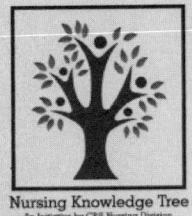

Practical Record Book of

Community Health Nursing

for Post Basic BSc Nursing Students

(As per the Syllabus of Indian Nursing Council for Post Basic BSc)

Indu Rathore MSc (CHN)

Assistant Professor
Murari Lal Memorial School and College of Nursing
Solan, Himachal Pradesh, India

Foreword

Sushma Kumari Saini

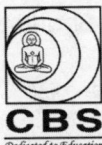

CBS
Dedicated to Education

CBS Publishers & Distributors Pvt Ltd

• New Delhi • Bengaluru • Chennai • Kochi • Kolkata • Lucknow
• Mumbai • Hyderabad • Nagpur • Patna • Pune • Vijayawada

Practical Record Book of

Community Health Nursing

for Post Basic BSc Nursing Students

ISBN: 978-93-86827-06-7

Copyright © Author and Publishers

Reprint: 2022
First Edition: 2018

Published by **Satish Kumar Jain** and produced by **Varun Jain** for

CBS Publishers & Distributors Pvt Ltd

4819/XI Prahlad Street, 24 Ansari Road, Daryaganj, New Delhi 110 002, India.
Ph: +91-11-23289259, 23266861, 23266867   Website: www.cbspd.com
Fax: 011-23243014
e-mail: delhi@cbspd.com; cbspubs@airtelmail.in.

Corporate Office: 204 FIE, Industrial Area, Patparganj, Delhi 110 092
Ph: +91-11-4934 4934   Fax: 4934 4935
e-mail: feedback@cbspd.com; bhupesharora@cbspd.com

Branches

- **Bengaluru:** Seema House 2975, 17th Cross, K.R. Road, Banasankari 2nd Stage, Bengaluru 560 070, Karnataka
  Ph: +91-80-26771678/79   Fax: +91-80-26771680   e-mail: bangalore@cbspd.com
- **Chennai:** 7, Subbaraya Street, Shenoy Nagar, Chennai 600 030, Tamil Nadu
  Ph: +91-44-26680620, 26681266   Fax: +91-44-42032115   e-mail: chennai@cbspd.com
- **Kochi:** 68/1534, 35, 36-Power House Road, Opp. KSEB, Cochin-682018, Kochi, Kerala
  Ph: +91-484-4059061-65   Fax: +91-484-4059065   e-mail: kochi@cbspd.com
- **Kolkata:** 6/B, Ground Floor, Rameswar Shaw Road, Kolkata-700 014, West Bengal
  Ph: +91-33-22891126, 22891127, 22891128   e-mail: kolkata@cbspd.com
- **Lucknow:** Basement, Khushnuma Complex, 7-Meerabai Marg, (Behind Jawahar Bhawan), Lucknow-226001, Uttar Pradesh
  Ph: +0522-4000032   e-mail: tiwari.lucknow@cbspd.com
- **Mumbai:** PWD Shed, Gala No. 25/26, Ramchandra Bhatt Marg, Next to J.J. Hospital Gate No. 2, Opp. Union Bank of India, Noor Baug, Mumbai-400009
  Ph: +91-22-66661880/89   Fax: +91-22-24902342   e-mail: mumbai@cbspd.com

Representatives

- **Hyderabad**   +91-9885175004
- **Pune**   +91-9623451994
- **Patna**   +91-9334159340
- **Vijayawada**   +91-9000660880

Printed at:

Dedicated to

Almighty God

My Family
and
Dear Students
who have been inspiration for me at every step of my life.

From Publisher's Desk

"Gaining knowledge is the first step to wisdom. Sharing it is the first step to humanity."

The above mentioned lines form the foundation stone of CBS publishers and Distributors Pvt Ltd, the flag bearer in medical publishing. Headquartered in New Delhi, the national capital of India, CBS was established in the year 1972 and it has expanded its roots to grow as a pioneer in the field of medical publishing in Asia. CBS is one of the largest and the fastest growing publishers of medical books in Southeast Asia. We are partners in the education of undergraduate and postgraduate students for we believe in nurturing the brains of medicos since the beginning of their careers in medicine. CBS joins the hands with the medical students as their first choice since the very moment they enter the college with BD Chaurasia's Human Anatomy and CC Chatterjee's Human Physiology. CBS is the proud owner of many bestselling titles like OP Ghai's Textbook of Pediatrics, Manipal's Surgery, KD Chatterjee's Textbook of Parasitology, and the list goes on. CBS has successfully partnered in sculpting the careers of millions of medicos across the world.

Since establishment of "CBS Nursing Knowledge Tree" last year we have published many successful titles in the field of nursing and we have proved ourselves in the nursing fraternity in providing Quality Education.

Vision and Mission of CBS Nursing Knowledge Tree

CBS Nursing Knowledge Tree is conceptualized with a vision of being the first of its kind to bring the best quality books for education of Nurses. Keeping in mind the changing trends in the Nursing Education, we at CBS have taken up a mission to bring student-friendly and syllabus-based books written by Subject Experts from PAN India without compromising on the Quality of content and presenting it in a Unique manner.

Foundation Stones of CBS Nursing Knowledge Tree

- **Strong editorial support by the leading subject experts and faculties in Nursing from PAN India.** Every manuscript/proposal that is received is critically reviewed by our Editorial Board at various levels to ensure the Quality of content. A book is published only after all the parameters in our process management are satisfied.

- **Special care taken to publish Plagiarism-free matter.** With the copyright laws being highly strict these days, we at CBS are paying extra attention at various stages of publishing a book to crosscheck and avoid any copyright infringement.

- **Books authored by Subject Experts and Senior Faculties all over India.** Every title owned by CBS Nursing Knowledge Tree is written by the senior-most faculties and subject masters from every nook and corner of the country to provide them a bigger platform to share their knowledge and experience amongst budding nursing fraternity.

- **All the books developed as per INC syllabus and needs of the students without compromising on the Quality of the content.** Often students complain that some books are either not covering the complete syllabus or have too much content as compared to the syllabus. In this series, extra care is being taken to develop books strictly as per INC syllabus in the most student-friendly manner.

- **All books being reviewed by Top-notch faculties and Subject Experts to maintain high standards of Quality.** Every title goes through tough grilling regarding the content and the overall presentation by various top subject experts as reviewers. This ensures that only the Quality content gets published.

- **Best International standard layouts for every book.** Every title in CBS Nursing Knowledge Tree is designed and formatted in the best layouts of international standards because we strongly believe that every book deserves to be treated the Best!

- **Additional and Unique features given with every title.** Every title is accompanied by one or the other additional feature to complement the learning of students like—*Workbook, DVD, Last Minute Revision Notes*. We have also included many features like *How to make Most out of this Book, Assess Yourself* that contains questions and MCQs and other special boxes according to the need of the content.

Let's Join Our Hands Together

We can only bring the change that we want to see in Nursing Education with the support and cooperation of leading faculties in all Nursing specialties. If you envision the same, we are happy to welcome you to our panel of contributors and reviewers and let's take up this mission together of creating a Change in Nursing Education.

We crave cooperation from all the students and faculties to provide their genuine feedback on the quality of the books and how we can improve upon the deficiencies in future on the following email id: cbsvpdesk@yahoo.com . Constructive criticism with concrete suggestions for improvement for all our books will be highly appreciated.

Expanding Horizons

We are also highly active in attending various National Level Conferences and Meets organized by various Nursing Societies. We are keenly working to expand our horizons of associations by participating in conferences organized by **SOCHNI, ISPN, NRSI, ICMR, SOMI,** etc. every year. CBS has always been a forerunner and a big supporter of all National level Nursing Conferences. *If you have any National and State level conference proposals, we are happy to be the part of these conferences.*

Being Social is Our Aspiration

In this era of Social Media, we are happy being social as well by bringing you our Facebook page **facebook.com/ cbsnursingtree** of "CBS Nursing Knowledge Tree" to expand our reach to the maximum people in Nursing. It is a platform purely dedicated to bring the important aspects and latest updates and developments in various domains and fields of Nursing. It will be our privilege if you could connect with us and share your knowledge and experiences as well on our Facebook page.

I would like to invite all the readers to come and join us on our facebook page and share some input, information and literature.

With this vision and above features we are happy to announce the release of Practical Record Book of Community Health Nursing for Post Basic BSc Nursing Students by Indu Rathore!

Bhupesh Arora
Vice President-Publishing and Marketing
(NURSING Division)
CBS Publishers and Distributors (Delhi) Pvt. Ltd.
Email: bhupesharora@cbspd.com
Mobile: (+91) 9555590180

Foreword

Community Health Nurses provide health care services to communities and improve their care accessibility. Key responsibilities of a community health nurse include: Identifying risk factors, improving access to services for under-served communities, promoting health care programs, providing direct care and screening services, educating people how to manage their conditions, performing immunizations, and ensuring maternal and child care. To fulfill these important roles, it is important for nursing students to learn skill in all these fields for which a comprehensive practical record book is very essential. I want to congratulate Ms Indu Rathore, Assistant Professor, Community Health Nursing, MLM School and College of Nursing, Solan (Himachal Pradesh) for bringing out such a comprehensive *Practical Record Book of Community Health Nursing for Post Basic BSc Nursing Students*.

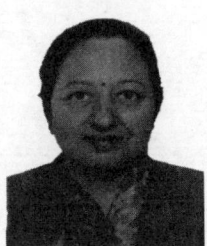

I personally liked the presentation of the book. It provides simple and systematic record book for undergraduate students. The BSc Nursing (Post Basic) students guided by their teachers in various aspects are expected to maintain quality and standard for community experience based on requirements, which were established for every college of nursing. This record book will benefit the Community Health Nursing (CHN) students in gaining practical skills in documenting community profile, family care study, family nursing care plan, health and nutrition assessment of different age groups. It provides enough space for recording different procedures, health teaching, practice teaching and visits to different health agencies. Enriched with reference notes, family folder and community survey proforma it inculcates better understanding of the practical aspects of CHN among nursing students. It also acts as guide for nursing teachers to teach and evaluate different aspects of community health nursing.

Annexures given at the end of the book is a unique feature of this book. This gives a quick reference of different laboratory tests normal values, nutritive values for commonly used food items in India and recommended dietary allowances for various categories. For teachers, it has given sample evaluation proformas to evaluate each practical skill of student. Author has covered all the practical aspects of community health nursing in very easy to understandable manner. A great deal of effort has been put into the format of the book to make it more user friendly. The entire book is prepared according to the current concepts of community health nursing. Upholds the latest syllabus and regulations of Indian Nursing Council.

I am sure this book will be proved as a boon for the nursing students and help them in strengthening their education, training and skill in performing their duties in implementing primary health care.

Sushma Kumari Saini

PhD (Public Administration), MSc Nursing (CHN)
Lecturer, National Institute of Nursing Education
PGIMER, Chandigarh, India

Preface

This Record Book is designed according to the community health nursing practical requirements of post basic BSc nursing students. Its main aim is to provide systematic, meaningful and comprehensive record of various activities and procedures carried out in a community setting. The record book is developed and updated according to latest syllabus prescribed by Indian Nursing Council, New Delhi.

The record book is prepared in a view to develop the standard format for conducting and writing the reports on community profile, family care study, family nursing care plans, health assessments of various age groups, health education plans, procedures or demonstrations using a standardized bag technique, A-V aid preparation, organization or participation in activities/clinics/camps, group projects, family folders and observation or orientation visits at health and welfare agencies. Further the evaluation proforma have been provided to maintain uniformity while evaluating nursing student's performance by the supervisors.

The special efforts have been taken to simplify the work and save time of supervisors or clinical instructors as well as nursing students. This record book serves as a valuable resource of logical, reliable and self-instructional formats to fulfill the community health nursing field requirements.

I hope that this record book will help the Post Basic BSc Nursing Students to gain knowledge and acquire competencies in community health nursing practice. I look forward for the valuable suggestions and reviews to make it more effective.

Indu Rathore

Acknowledgements

"When performance exceeds ambition, the overlap is called success"

First and foremost, I would like to thank the Lord for his grace and abundant blessings that I could complete this record book on time.

I express my sincere gratitude and I feel indebted to extend thanks to Mrs Shashi Sharma, Principal, MLM School and College of Nursing, Solan (Himachal Pradesh). Without her guidance and persistent help this work would not have been possible.

I am thankful to Mrs Neeti Sharma, Vice-principal, MLM School and College of Nursing, Solan (HP) for helping me to form valid concepts for this record book. Their deep insight and experience has given the present shape to my project.

I gratefully acknowledge Mr Nimit Gupta, Director, MLM School and College of Nursing, Solan (HP) for providing valuable assets, infrastructure and resources throughout the writing period. He has all along been considerate, helpful and cordial despite his hectic schedule and official commitments.

I gratefully acknowledge the contribution all faculty members of MLM School and College of Nursing, Solan (HP) for their help and innumerable suggestions.

I will ever remain indebted to my family members—Father (Mr Shyam Babu Rathore), mother (Mrs Savitri Rathore), brother (Paurush) and sister (Neha), who always stood beside me through my tough times. They have been behind the scene, patiently encouraging and inspiring me.

Finally and perhaps most importantly, I would like to express my special appreciation to **Mr Satish Kumar Jain** (Chairman) and **Mr Varun Jain** (Managing Director), M/s CBS Publishers and Distributors Pvt Ltd for their wholehearted support in publication of this book. I also thank **Mr Bhupesh Arora**, (Vice President) Publishing and Marketing Nursing Division for providing me the platform to share knowledge and an opportunity to add to the existing knowledge of this field. I personally thank Mr Anubhav Puri for being with me from the beginning till end of this project.

I would like to thank Dr Mrinalini Bakshi (Sr. Content Developer and Editor) for her editorial support on this project. I personally thank Ms Nitasha Arora (Project Manager), Ms Neetu Jindal (Asst Production Manager), Mr Nitish K Dubey (Sr Editor) and all the production team members Mr Ashutosh Pathak, Mr Bunty Kashyap, Mr Phool Kumar, Mr Chaman Lal, Mr Prakash Gaur, Mr Prabhat Ranjan, Ms Tahira Parveen, Ms Babita Verma, Mr Raju Sharma, Mr Vikram Chaudhary and Manoj Chaudhary for devoting laborious hours in designing and type-setting of the book.

I extend my gratitude to all my students for their cooperation. My sincere thanks to all those who had directly and indirectly helped me in this endeavor.

Syllabus for Post Basic BSc Nursing

COMMUNITY HEALTH NURSING

PRACTICAL

Placement: Second Year

Time: 240 Hours

Areas	Duration	Practicum
Community Health Nursing (Urban/Rural)	240 Hours	❑ Each student will prepare a community profile. ❑ The students will be allotted families for gaining experience in identifying family health needs, health counseling and guidance and family budgeting for optimum health. ❑ The students will participate in the activities of primary health centre, Sub-centre, MCH Centre. ❑ Visits will be made to selected health and welfare agencies, water purification plant and sewage disposal plant, infectious disease hospital. ❑ Conduct health educational programmes for individual/groups/community.

Contents

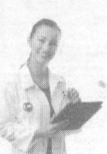

Student Profile

Paste Your Recent Passport Size Photograph in Uniform

Name of the Student: _____

Registration No./Enrolment No.: _____

Session/Batch: _____

Name of the Institution: _____

Name of the University: _____

Signature of Student

Date _____

Signature of HOD

Date _____

Signature of Principal

Date _____

Signature of:

Internal Examiner

Date _____

External Examiner

Date _____

Supplementary Examination

Signature of:

Internal Examiner

Date _____

External Examiner

Date _____

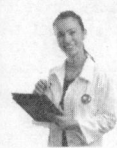

1. Community Profile
(Based on Community Identification and Vital Statistics Survey)

INTRODUCTION OF COMMUNITY

General Information

Village/Area Name: _____

Panchayat: _____

Block: _____

Tehsil/Taluka: _____

District: _____

Total population: _____

Total Families: _____

Nearby Health Care Facilities [Name and its distance (in km) from the community area]

District Hospital: _____

Government Maternity Hospital (if any): _____

Mission Hospital (if any): _____

Total Private Hospitals: _____

Sub Center: _____

Primary Health Center: _____

Community Health Center: _____

Indigenous Medicine (Hospital/Clinic/Dispensary)

- Ayurveda: _____
- Yoga: _____
- Naturopathy: _____
- Unani: _____
- Siddha: _____
- Homeopathy: _____
- If other, Specify: _____

Non-Governmental Organizations/Voluntary Health Organizations

- Orphan Age Children _____
- Physically Challenged _____
- Visually Challenged _____

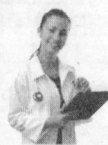

- Mentally Challenged _____
- Hearing Challenged _____
- Women _____
- Elderly _____
- Youth Welfare _____
- Other _____

Social Agencies

- Post Office _____
- Bank _____
- Police Station _____

Religious Place

- Temple _____
- Mosque _____
- Gurudwara _____
- Church _____
- If Others, Specify _____

Education Facilities

Government

- Anganwadis _____
- Balwadis _____
- Primary School _____
- Elementary School _____
- Secondary School _____
- Senior Secondary School _____
- UG Institutions _____
- PG Institutions _____

Private

- Primary School _____
- Elementary School _____
- Secondary School _____
- Senior Secondary School _____
- UG Institutions _____
- PG institutions _____

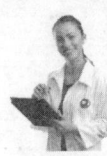

Recreation Facilities

- Common Market Place _____
- Playgrounds _____
- Public Gardens _____
- Cinema Halls _____
- Clubs _____
- Public Library _____
- Fairs _____
- Festivals _____

Communication Facilities

- Post Office _____
- Public Telephone Booths _____
- Computer Center with Internet Facility _____
- Traditional Media (Puppets, Folk Dance etc.) _____

Transport Facilities

- Railway Station _____
- Bus Stand _____
- Auto Stand _____
- Taxi Stand _____
- Airport _____

Facilities for the Disposal of Dead Bodies

_____

_____

_____

_____

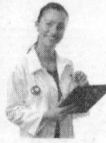

SOCIO-DEMOGRAPHIC DATA

N =

S. No.		Socio-demographic Characteristics	n (%)
1.	Age Group	Infant (1–12 months) Under Five Children (1–5 years) School Going (6–12 years) Adolescent (13–17 years) Early Adult (18–45 years) Late Adult (46–59 years) Geriatric (60 years and above)	
2.	Sex	Male Female Transgender	
3.	Religion*	Hindu Muslim Christian Sikh Others, Specify _____	
4.	Caste	General OBC SC ST	
5.	Education**	Illiterate Able to read and write Primary Up to 8th class Up to 10th Up to 12th Graduate Post Graduate PhD/M.Phil Others, Specify _____	
6.	Marital status	Married Single/Unmarried Widow	
7.	Type of family	Nuclear Joint Separated	
8.	Family Size	2–4 5–8 9 and above	
9.	Occupation	Employed—Government Job Private Job Unemployed Retired Daily wage workers Homemaker	
10.	Total Family Income (₹)	Up to 10000 10000–20000 20000 and above	

*Other religion _____   **Other educational qualification _____

PHYSICAL CHARACTERISTICS OF AREA (MAP)

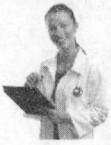

Keys

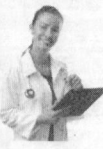

HOUSING STANDARDS

N =

S. No.	Characteristics		n (%)
1.	Ownership of house	Rent	
		Own	
2.	Type of house	Pucca	
		Semi pucca	
		Katcha	
3.	Number of living room per House	1–2	
		3–4	
		4 and above	
4.	Bathroom	Not available	
		Available - Own	
		Public	
		Hygiene - Hygienic	
		Unhygienic	
5.	Latrine	Not available	
		Available - Own	
		Public	
		Hygiene - Hygienic	
		Unhygienic	
6.	Electricity	Not available	
		Available	
7.	Water Supply*	Tap	
		Well	
		Lake/pond	
		Others, Specify _____	
8.	Kitchen **	Separate	
		Corner of the room	
		Others, Specify _____	
9.	Type of fuel used***	LPG	
		Electricity	
		Kerosene	
		Wood	
		Others, Specify _____	

*Other water supply source _____ **Other kitchen _____

***Other fuel used _____

HOUSING ENVIRONMENT AND SANITATION

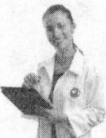

N =

S. No.	Characteristics		n (%)
1.	Modern sanitation facility	Drainage system	
		Sewage system	
2.	Drainage System	Closed	
		Open	
3.	Refuse Disposal	Open dumping	
		Composting	
		Burning	
		Municipality collection/community bins	
4.	Domestic animal*	Not present	
		Present - Dog	
		Cat	
		Buffalo	
		Cow	
		Goat	
		Others, Specify _____	
5.	Cattle shed (for the house with domestic animal)	Yes	
		No	
6.	Domestic birds/poultry**	Not present	
		Present - Hen/Cock	
		Parrot	
		Others, Specify _____	
7.	Poultry shed/cage (for the house with poultry)	Yes	
		No	
8.	Rodents	Not present	
		Yes - Rat	
		Others, Specify _____	
9.	Insects	Not present	
		Yes - Mosquitoes	
		Flies	
		Ticks	
		Others, Specify _____	
10.	Street animals	Not present	
		Yes - Dogs	
		Cats	
		Cows	
		Others, Specify _____	

*Other domestic animals _____

**Other domestic birds _____

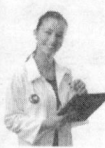

FAMILY PLANNING STATUS

N =

S. No.	Methods adopted for Family Planning		n (%)
1.	Temporary Methods	Condoms	
		Oral Contraceptive Pills(OCP)	
		Copper-T (Cu-T)	
		Injectables	
		Sub dermal Implants	
2.	Permanent Methods	Tubectomy	
		Vasectomy	
3.	Not adopting any family planning method		

COMMON HEALTH PROBLEMS

N =

S. No.	Health Problems	n (%)
1.	Communicable Diseases	
2.	Non- communicable Diseases	
3.	Nutritional Problems	
4.	Mental Health Problems	
5.	Acute Problems	
6.	Chronic Problems	

VITAL STATISTICS

1. Crude Birth Rate

$$\text{Crude Birth Rate} = \frac{\text{No. of live birth during the year}}{\text{Estimated mid-year population}} \times 1000$$

Crude Birth Rate = _____

2. Crude Death Rate

$$\text{Crude Death Rate} = \frac{\text{No. of deaths during the year}}{\text{Estimated mid-year population}} \times 1000$$

Crude Death Rate = _____

3. Infant Mortality Rate

$$\text{Infant Mortality Rate} = \frac{\text{No. of deaths under one year of age}}{\text{Total live births in the same year}} \times 1000$$

Infant Mortality Rate = _____

4. Neonatal Mortality Rate

$$\text{Neonatal Mortality Rate} = \frac{\text{No. of deaths of children less than 28 days in a year}}{\text{Total live births in the same year}} \times 1000$$

Neonatal Mortality Rate = _____

5. Still Birth Rate

$$\text{Still Birth Rate} = \frac{\text{No. of still births in a year}}{\text{Total live births and still births in the same year}} \times 1000$$

Still Birth Rate = _____

6. Maternal Mortality Rate

$$\text{Maternal Mortality Rate} = \frac{\text{Total No. of female deaths due to complications of pregnancy, child birth or within 42 days of delivery during a given year}}{\text{Total number of live births in the same year}} \times 1000$$

Maternal Mortality Rate = _____

7. General Fertility Rate

$$\text{General Fertility Rate} = \frac{\text{No. of live births in area during the year}}{\text{Mid-year female population age group (15–49) in the same year}} \times 1000$$

General Fertility Rate = _____

ONGOING COMMUNITY HEALTH PROGRAMMES

(Communicable/non-communicable diseases/others)

ONGOING SOCIAL WELFARE/HEALTH SCHEMES

Physically/Visually/Mentally/Hearing Challenged

_____

_____

_____

Women (Antenatal/Postnatal/Widow)

_____

_____

_____

Children

_____

_____

_____

Adolescent Girls

_____

_____

_____

BPL Families

_____

_____

_____

Elderly

_____

_____

_____

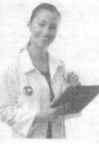

LIST OF COMMUNITY LEADERS

Department	Designation	Name	Address	Contact number
FORMAL LEADERS				
Political system	MLA			
	MP			
	Representative of women			
	Representative of SC/ST			
	Trade Union Leaders			
Gram panchayat	President (Pradhan/Sarpanch)			
	Vice President/Panchayat secretary (Uppradhan/Upsarpanch)			
Ward	Ward member (councillor)			
Health	Health Worker (Female)			
	Health Worker (Male)			
	Anganwadi worker			
INFORMAL LEADERS				
School	School Teacher			
Society	Social Worker			
	Retired person			
Others				

IDENTIFIED COMMUNITY HEALTH NEEDS

_____
_____
_____
_____
_____
_____
_____
_____
_____
_____
_____
_____
_____
_____
_____
_____
_____
_____
_____

COMMUNITY HEALTH ACTION PLAN

Health Needs Identified	Planning/Nursing Interventions

Signature of Student

Signature of Supervisor

15

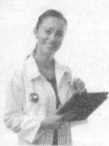

2. Family Care Study

IDENTIFICATION DATA

Name of the Area: _____

Name of Informant: _____

Relationship with Head of Family: _____

Age/Sex: _____

House No.: _____

Date of Starting: _____

Date of Ending: _____

INTRODUCTION OF THE FAMILY

General Information

Name of Head of the Family: _____

Address: _____

Nearby Sub-center/PHC/CHC/District Hospital: _____

Religion—Hindu/Muslims/Sikh/Christian/Others: _____

Caste—GEN/SC/ST/OBC: _____

Occupation of the head of the family—Unemployed/Government/Private Job/Self-Employed/Daily Wage Worker/ Homemaker/Others: _____

Language known—Hindi/English/Others: _____

Family Size (Total Members): _____

Family Type—Nuclear/Joint: _____

Ownership of House—Own/Rented: _____

Monthly Family Income—₹: _____

Family income per Capita—₹: _____

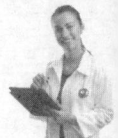

FAMILY COMPOSITION AND CHARACTERISTICS

S. No.	Name of the family members	Relationship with head of the family	Date of birth/sex (Male-M/Female-F/Transgender-T)	Marital status (Unmarried/married)	Educational status	Occupation	Monthly income (₹)	Dietary habits (veg/non-veg)	Addiction (smoking/alcohol/drugs/others)	Health status (healthy/unhealthy)
1.										
2.										
3.										
4.										
5.										
6.										
7.										
8.										

Key

Family Tree/Genogramme

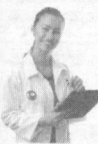

AVAILABILITY OF HEALTH CARE/SOCIAL/EDUCATIONAL FACILITIES

Facilities	Yes/No (If yes, specify name and distance from the house)
Nearby Health care facilities	
District hospital	
Government maternity hospital (if any)	
Private hospitals	
Sub center	
Primary health center	
Community health center	
Indigenous medicine (hospital/clinic/dispensary)	
• Ayurveda	
• Yoga	
• Naturopathy	
• Unani	
• Siddha	
• Homeopathy	
• If other, specify	
Non-Governmental Organizations/Voluntary Health Organizations	
• Orphan age children	
• Physically challenged	
• Visually challenged	
• Mentally challenged	
• Hearing challenged	
• Women	
• Elderly	
• Youth welfare	
• Other	
Social Agencies	
• Post office	
• Bank	
• Police station	
Education facilities	
Government	
• Anganwadis	
• Balwadis	
• Primary school	
• Elementary school	
• Secondary school	
• Senior secondary school	
• UG Institutions	
• PG institutions	
Private	
• Primary school	
• Elementary school	
• Secondary school	
• Senior secondary school	
• UG Institutions	
• PG institutions	

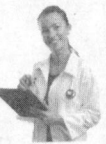

AVAILABILITY OF RECREATION/COMMUNICATION/TRANSPORT/RELIGIOUS FACILITIES

Facilities	Yes/No (If yes, specify name and distance from the house)
Recreation facilities	
• Nearby market	
• Playgrounds	
• Public Gardens	
• Cinema halls	
• Clubs	
• Public Library	
• Fairs	
• Festivals	
Communication facilities	
• Telephone connection	
• Mobile phone	
• Internet facility	
• Letters	
Transport facilities	
• Bus	
• Auto rickshaw	
• Taxi	
• Four wheeler	
• Two wheeler	
• Train	
• Airway	
Religious places	
• Temple	
• Mosque	
• Gurudwara	
• Church	

Sketch of House

(Draw a sketch of the house showing location of rooms, doors, windows, entrance of the house, drinking water source, toilet, kitchen)

Key

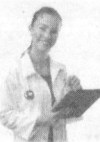

HOUSING STANDARDS AND ENVIRONMENTAL CONDITIONS

Characteristic	Parameters
Type of house	Pucca/Semi pucca/Katcha
Site	Elevated from surroundings/depressed from surroundings
Total number of living room	1/2/3/4/5/6/7/8/_____
Space per person	Adequate (1 room -2 persons, 2 rooms -3 persons, 3 rooms – 5 persons, 4 rooms -7 persons, 5 or more rooms - 10 persons (additional 2 for each further room Inadequate (if above criteria is not fulfilled)
Ventilation	Adequate (doors and windows facing each other in each room) Inadequate (doors and windows not facing each other in each room)
Bathroom Hygiene	Not available/If available—Own/Public Hygienic/Unhygienic
Wall	Plastered or Cemented/Tiled/Wooden/Unplastered/Mud//Others, specify _____

Roof
  Height
  Painting
	
	Less than 10 feet/More than 10 feet
	Light colored/Dark colored

Day light	Adequate (Able to read the small fonts of newspaper inside the room during the day without any artificial lighting) Inadequate (Not able to read the small fonts of newspaper inside the room during the day without any artificial lighting)
Latrine Hygiene	Not available/If available—Own/Public Hygienic/Unhygienic
Electricity	Not available/Available
Drinking water supply	Tap/Well/Lake/Pond/Others, specify _____
Kitchen	Separate/Corner of the room/Others, specify _____
Type of fuel used	LPG/Electricity/Kerosene/Wood/Others, specify _____
Open space around the house	Absent/Present
Stagnant water around the house	Absent/Present
Street road	Tar/Cement/Mud/Others
Street light	Absent/Present

Modern sanitation facility
  Drainage system
  Sewage system
	
	Yes/No
	Yes/No

Drainage System	Closed/Open
Refuse Disposal	Open dumping/Composting/Burning/Municipality collection/Community bins/Others, specify _____
Domestic animal	Absent/If present—Dog/Cow/Buffalo/Goat/Camel/Others, specify _____
Separate cattle shed (for the house with domestic animals)	Yes/No
Domestic birds/Poultry	Absent/If present—Hen/Cock/Parrot/Others, specify _____
Separate poultry shed/cage (for the house with domestic birds)	Yes/No
Rodents	Absent/If present—Rat/Others, specify _____
Street animals	Absent/If present—Dogs/Cats/Cows/Others, specify _____
Insect vectors	Absent/If present—Mosquitoes/Flies/Ticks/Others, specify _____

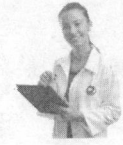

SOCIOECONOMIC STATUS

Social class/Socioeconomic status (according to rural/urban socioeconomic scale, Refer: to Annexures)

VULNERABLE/TARGET GROUPS IN THE FAMILY

Total eligible couples _____   Children (0–1 years) _____   Adolescent Girls _____

Total postnatal mothers _____   Children (1–3 years) _____   Elderly (above 60 years) _____

Total antenatal mothers _____   Children (3–5 years) _____   Other, specify _____

MONTHLY FAMILY BUDGET

Income			Expenditure		
Sources	**Income (In ₹)**	**Income (In Percentage)**	**Sources**	**Expenditure (In ₹)**	**Expenditure (In Percentage)**
Salary			House Rent		
Rent			Education		
Agriculture			Food		
Animals			Fuel (LPG)		
Pension			Fuel (Petrol/Diesel)		
Stipend			Clothing		
Part time business			Entertainment		
Others			Electricity		
			Water		
			Property Taxes		
			Telephone/Internet		
			Transportation		
			Health		
			Festival		
			Saving		
			Insurance		
			Others		
Total (₹)			**Total (₹)**		

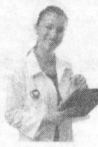

FAMILY DIETARY PATTERN

Food group	Food item	Food consumption (Yes/No)	Frequency of consumption (servings per day or per week)	Method/Form of food preparation (boiling/steaming/raw/ pressure cooking/ frying/germination etc.)	Method of food storage at home (Hygienic-H/ Unhygienic-U)
Energy giving foods	Rice				
	Wheat				
	Tubers				
	Edible oil				
	Ghee				
	Butter				
Body building foods	Meat				
	Fish				
	Poultry				
	Eggs				
	Pulses				
Protective foods	Vegetables				
	Fruits				
	Milk & milk products				
Beverages	Tea				
	Coffee				
	Water				
Others	Junk food				

SOCIOCULTURAL ASPECTS

Menstruation _____

_____

_____

_____

_____

_____

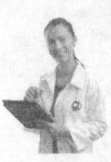

Antenatal Care _____

_____

_____

_____

_____

_____

Child Birth _____

_____

_____

_____

_____

_____

Postnatal Care _____

_____

_____

_____

_____

_____

Care of Sick _____

_____

_____

_____

_____

_____

Food Consumption _____

_____

_____

_____

_____

_____

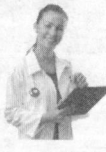

FAMILY PLANNING STATUS (ELIGIBLE COUPLE)

S. No.	Name of the eligible couple (Mr. _____ Mrs. _____)	Age (yrs.)/ Sex (Male-M Female-F)	Family Planning Practice a) Yes b) No	If yes, then								
				Temporary Family Planning Method					Permanent Family Planning Method		Month and year of adoption/ Duration of use	
				Condom	Oral pills	Copper-T	Inject able	Implant	Tubectomy	Vasectomy		
1.												
2.												
3.												
4.												

IMMUNIZATION STATUS

Age Group	Weeks/ Months/Years	Current Vaccine Under UIP (2017)	Child Name/Vaccines/Date of administration (D.O.A.)					
			Child -1 _____		Child -2 _____		Child -3 _____	
			Vaccines	D.O.A.	Vaccines	D.O.A.	Vaccines	D.O.A.
Infant	At birth	BCG, OPV-0, Hep-B birth dose						
	6 weeks	OPV-1, Rota-1, Pentavalent-1, IPV-1, PCV-1						
	10 weeks	OPV-1, Rota-2, Pentavalent-2						
	14 weeks	OPV-3, Rota-3, Pentavalent-3, IPV-2, PCV-2						
	9 months	MR/Measles-1, Vit-A*, JE-1#, PCV-Booster						
Under five Children	16-24 months	DPT-Booster-1, OPV-Booster, MR/Measles-2, JE-2#						
School Going	5-6 Years	DPT-Booster -2						
Adolescent	10 years	TT-1						
	16 years	TT-2						
Pregnancy		TT-1						
		TT-2						

*Vitamin A to be given every 6 months till five years of age and a separate chart is given below for documentation. #JE vaccine given in selected districts. **BCG:** Bacillus Calmette-Guerin; **Pentavalent [DPT:** diphtheria-pertussis-tetanus; **Hep B:** Hepatitis B; **Hib:**Haemophilus influenzae type b]; **JE:** Japanese Encephalitis; **MR/Measles/MMR:** Measles Mumps rubella; **OPV:** oral polio vaccine; **TT:** tetanus toxoid; **IPV:** inactivated poliovirus vaccine. **Rota-** Rotavirus vaccine, **PCV:** Pneumonia; Additional

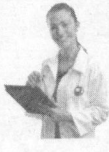

Age (in months) →		9	18	24	30	36	42	48	54	60
Dose →		1st	2nd	3rd	4th	5th	6th	7th	8th	9th
Vitamin-A Solution (D.O.A.)	Child-1 _____									
	Child-2 _____									
	Child-3 _____									

VITAL EVENTS IN THE FAMILY DURING THE LAST ONE YEAR

Birth (if any)

S. No.	Name	Date of Birth	Sex	Parents Name	Place of Birth	Birth registration-Yes/No
1.						
2.						
3.						

Death (if any)

S. No.	Name	Date of Death	Age/Sex	Cause of Death	Place of Death	Death registration-Yes/No
1.						
2.						
3.						

Marriage (if any)

S. No.	Name of the couple	Age		Date of marriage	Marriage registration-Yes/No
		Wife	Husband		
1.					
2.					
3.					

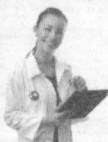

Family Health Profile

Instructions

1. Include all the available family members—elderly, adult woman, adult male, adolescent, antenatal, postnatal mother, newborn, children, physically challenged, sick, vulnerable or specific group as per assigned family health need.
2. Four complete proformas [including adults (2) & elderly (2)] are provided here. If not applicable leave them blank.
3. Twenty-four blank pages are provided to prepare the health profile of rest of the family members.
4. In these blank pages include family members identification data, health history, specific physical assessment, lab investigations, medications, diet chart, identified health needs/problems, and disease condition (book picture) etc.

1. ADULT

Name: _____ Age/Sex _____

Classification/Diagnosis: _____

BRIEF HISTORY

History of present complaints (character/onset/location/duration/severity pattern/associated factors/medication and treatment)

_____

_____

_____

_____

_____

_____

_____

_____

Past health (medical/surgical) history (problems at birth/infancy/childhood/immunization/adulthood (physical, mental, and psychological)/allergies (food/medication/others)/Chronic illness (e.g. hypertension, diabetes mellitus, heart, liver, renal disease etc./hereditary/communicable disease/any surgery and reason/other history)

_____

_____

_____

_____

_____

_____

_____

Menstrual History

Age at menarche: _____ yrs   **Menstruation:** Regular/irregular   **Length of cycle:** _____ days

Duration of blood flow: _____ days   LMP _____   Age at Menopause _____ yr

Dysmenorrhea: Present/absent   **Leucorrhea:** Present/absent   **Menorrhagia:** Present/absent

Marital History

Age at marriage _____ yrs   Duration of marriage _____ yrs

Consanguineous marriage—Yes/No   Relationship with spouse—satisfactory/unsatisfactory

Obstetric History

S. No	Year	Pregnancy (normal/ complicated)	Type of Delivery (Normal/Assisted/LSCS)	Place of Delivery (Hospital/ Home)	Delivery conducted by (Doctor/Nurse/ Dai/Other)	Alive/ Still borne	Sex	Birth-weight (in kg)	Present Condition (Alive/ dead)
1.									
2.									
3.									
4.									
5.									
6.									

Personal and Social History

Dietary pattern (veg/non-veg/lacto-ovo-vegetarian)/No. of meals per day/staple food/fasting habits

_____

_____

_____

_____

Bowel and bladder habit (regular/irregular, stool frequency and consistency)

_____

_____

_____

_____

Rest/sleep/activity/exercise/travel

_____

_____

_____

Occupation (type/working hours per day/work place stress/job satisfaction)

_____

_____

_____

_____

_____

Habits (alcohol/smoking/drugs/tobacco/chewing betel leaves)

_____

_____

_____

_____

_____

Leisure/recreational/religious/spiritual activities

_____

_____

_____

_____

_____

Relationship with family members/relatives/friends/others—satisfactory/unsatisfactory

_____

_____

_____

_____

_____

PHYSICAL EXAMINATION (put a tick (✓) mark wherever necessary or mention the finding in the provided space if needed)

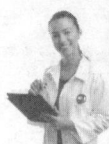

General Appearance

Consciousness: Conscious/semi-conscious/unconscious/confused

Posture: Normal/kyphosis/lordosis/scoliosis

Body built: Thin/moderate/obese

Nourishment: Well-nourished/under nourished

Activity: Active/dull/lethargic

Dress/grooming: Well-groomed/dirty

Gait (ability to walk/move): Normal/unsteady/any limp

Look: Normal/anxious/depressed/fear

Anthropometric Measurement

Weight: _____kg, Height: _____ cm, BMI (Quetelet's Index)_____[weight (kg)/height²(meter)]

Waist Circumference _____cm

Hip Circumference _____cm

Waist/Hip Ratio- _____ (normal < 0.85)

Vital Signs

Temperature -_____°C, Pulse-_____beats/m, Respiration _____breaths/m, BP _____ mm Hg,

Pain (5th vital sign)-absent/if present-onset/intensity/duration/type/location

_____

_____

_____

Skin Condition

Color: Normal/redness/flushing/cyanosis/jaundice/ pallor/pigmented/white patches

Texture: Smooth/soft/rough/dry/wrinkled/edematous

Lesions: Absent/macule/papule/vesicle/pustule/ulcer/scab

Temperature: Normal (warm)/cool/hot

Turgor (elasticity): Normal/decreased

_____

Head

Shape: Symmetrical/asymmetrical

Scalp: Normal/lesion/lump/infection/psoriasis

Hair: Colour: Normal/grey/white/artificial color

    Texture: Smooth/rough/dry/flaky/oily/thin

    Dandruff: Present/absent

    Alopecia: Present/absent

    Pediculosis: Present/absent

    Hygiene: Good/poor

Face

Shape: Symmetrical/asymmetrical

Color: Normal/pale/flushed

Edema: Present/absent

Movement: Normal/tics/tremors/fasciculation

Eyes

Eye	Right	Left
Discharge: Present/absent		
Eyebrows: Symmetrical/asymmetrical/absent		
Eyelids: Normal/edema/ptosis/entropion/ectropion		
Eyelashes: Normal/stye/infection		
Eyeball: Normal/protruded/sunken		
Sclera: Normal/jaundice/redness		
Conjunctiva: Normal/moist/pale/red/watery/purulent		
Pupils: Cloudy/dilated/constricted/reacting to light		
Vision: Normal/myopia/hyperopia		
Glasses/contact lens: Present/absent		

Ears

Ear	Right	Left
Shape: Symmetrical/asymmetrical with head		
External ear: Normal/discharge/earwax accumulation/pain/itching		
Auditory canal: Smooth/pink/redness/discharge/wax plug/lesion/foreign body		
Tympanic membrane: Intact/redness/swelling/perforated/bulging		
Gross Hearing: Normal/using hearing aid		

Nose

Discharge/crust: Present/absent

Nasal septum: Intact/perforated/deviation _____

Mucous membrane: Normal (moist & red)/dry/lesion/discharge/swollen/epistaxis

Polyp: Present/absent

Flaring: Present/absent

Mouth

Odor: Normal/foul smelling

Lips: Normal (pink, moist, smooth)/dry/cracked/cyanosis/swelling/redness/crust/cheilosis

Gums: Normal (pink and smooth)/swelling/bleeding/pus/gingivitis

Tongue/mucus: Normal (pink and moist)/pale/dry/coated/redness/lesion/swelling/glossitis

Teeth: Normal/poor alignment/missing/dental caries/plaque/discoloration _____

Tonsils: Normal (small, pink, symmetrical)/inflammation/enlarged/lesion/exudate

Throat and pharynx: Normal/redness/pus/lesion/exudate

29

contd…

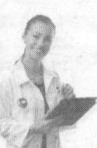

Neck

Lymph nodes (preauricular, parotid, postauricular, occipital, tonsillar, submaxillary, submental, anterior and deep cervical chain, posterior cervical, supraclavicular)- non-palpable/enlarge/tender

Thyroid gland: Normal (soft and elastic)/asymmetrical/enlarge/lump/bulging

Range of motion(flexion/extension/rotation): Symmetrical/asymmetrical neck with ROM

Chest

Shape/contour: Symmetrical/asymmetrical
Breathing pattern: Normal/unequal chest expansion/use of accessory muscles
Breath sounds: Normal/abnormal-wheezing/rhonchi/crackles/stridor/others _____
Sputum: Absent/if present, color/consistency _____
_____

Heart rate: Normal/fast/slow _____
Heart rhythm: Regular/irregular _____
Heart sounds: Normal/abnormal-murmur/others _____
_____

Female Breast

Breast	Right	Left
Size: Round/smooth/retraction/dimpling/lump/swollen/tender Shape: Symmetrical/asymmetrical		
Areola: Normal(moist, round)/dry Nipple: Everted/inversion/flat/cracked/crusted/discharge Axillary lymph nodes: Non-palpable/mobile/enlarge/tender Mass or lump: Absent/location/shape/size/consistency/tenderness _____		

Monthly Breast Self-Examination: Yes/No

Abdomen

Inspection
Shape: Symmetrical/asymmetrical/distension/observable mass/hernia/ascites/unusual pulsation
Color: Normal/white and silver lines (striae)
Skin: Normal/lesion/rashes/previous surgery scar/vascularity

Auscultation
Bowel sounds: Present/absent/frequency _____ movements/min

Palpation
Superficial palpation: Soft/pain/tenderness/mass _____
_____

Deep palpation (in all 4 quadrants for palpable organs): No organomegaly/pain/tenderness/palpable- liver/spleen/urinary bladder/appendix/inguinal hernia _____
Percussion: Presence of gas/fluid/mass (dullness)/liver margins _____

Extremities

Upper extremities: Right Left	Right	Left
Range of motion: Symmetrical/asymmetrical		
Fingers: Normal/polydactyly/syndactyly arachnodactyly/edema/tremors/nodules/crepitus/pain		
Nails		
Color: Pink/pale/cyanosis		
Shape: Normal (convex)/spoon-shaped/beau's lines/flat/clubbed		
Hygiene: Clean/dirty/long/short		

Capillary refill time.......seconds (Normal<3 seconds)

Lower Extremities	Right	Left
Range of motion: Symmetrical/asymmetrical Toe/foot: Normal/polydactyly/syndactyly/arachnodactyly/nodule/edema/pain/alignment/position/shape _____ _____		
Joint: Normal/warm/swollen/tender/painful		
Nails:		
Color: Pink/pale/cyanosis Shape: Normal (convex)/spoon-shaped/beau's lines/flat/clubbed Hygiene: Clean/dirty/long/short Varicose veins: Present/absent		

Rectum

Rectum and anus: Normal/hemorrhoids/fissures/polyp/ulcer/lesion/rashes/redness/bleeding
Stool: Color/odor/consistency _____
_____

Sacrococcygeal Area: Swelling/redness/dimpling or hair
Bowel pattern: Regular/irregular

Urinary Bladder

Bladder pattern: Normal/burning micturition/dribbling of urine while working or coughing
Urine: Color/odor/frequency _____

contd...

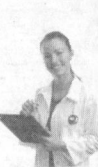

Genitals

Female Genitalia

Mons pubis: Normal/lesions/redness/edema
Labia majora: Normal/lesions/redness/edema
Perineum: Normal/lesions/redness/edema
Vagina: Normal/redness/lesion/discharge/pain _____
Urethra: Normal/discharge/redness/swelling _____
Inguinal lymph nodes: Normal/enlarge/tender/palpable

Male genitalia

Scrotum: Symmetrical/asymmetrical/lesions/redness/swelling/
pain/discharge/mass _____
_____
Penis: Normal/tenderness/pain/discharge
Foreskin: Intact/retractable/lesions
Location of urinary orifice: Normal/ventral/dorsal surface
Urethra: Normal/discharge/redness/swelling
Inguinal lymph nodes: Normal/enlarge/tender/palpable
Inguinal hernia: Absent/present
Monthly Testicular Self-Examination: Yes/No

LAB INVESTIGATIONS

S. No.	Date/time	Investigation	Patient value	Normal value	Remarks

MEDICATIONS

S. No.	Name and action	Dose/route/frequency	Indication	Side-effects

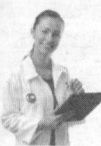

DIETARY PATTERN (24 HOURS RECALL)

Meal Time	Food item	Major Content	Quantity	Calories (kcal)	Carbohy-drate(g)	Protein (g)	Fat (g)	Iron (mg)	Calcium (mg)
Breakfast (__am)									
Midmorning (__am)									
Lunch (__pm)									
Evening Tea (__pm)									
Dinner (__pm)									
Bed time (__pm)									
Total									
Recommended Daily Values									
Deficient (–)/Excess (+)									

MODIFIED DIET PLAN

Meal Time	Food item	Major Content	Quantity	Calories (kcal)	Carbohy-drate(g)	Protein (g)	Fat (g)	Iron (mg)	Calcium (mg)
Breakfast (__am)									
Midmorning (__am)									
Lunch (__pm)									
Evening Tea (__pm)									
Dinner (__pm)									
Bed time (__pm)									
Total									
Recommended Daily Values									
Deficient (–)/Excess (+)									

Identified Health Problems/Needs

_____

_____

_____

_____

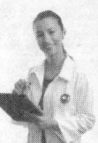

DISEASE CONDITION

(Book picture/comparison with available literature)

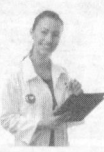

2. ADULT

Name: _____ Age/Sex _____

Classification/Diagnosis: _____

BRIEF HISTORY

History of present complaints (character/onset/location/duration/severity pattern/associated factors/medication and treatment)

_____

_____

_____

_____

_____

_____

_____

_____

_____

_____

_____

_____

_____

Past health (medical/surgical) history (problems at birth/infancy/childhood/immunization/adulthood (physical, mental, and psychological)/allergies (food/medication/others)/Chronic illness (e.g. hypertension, diabetes mellitus, heart, liver, renal disease etc./hereditary/communicable disease/any surgery and reason/other history)

_____

_____

_____

_____

_____

_____

_____

_____

_____

_____

Menstrual History

Age at menarche: _____ yrs **Menstruation:** Regular/irregular **Length of cycle:** _____ days

Duration of blood flow: _____ days LMP _____ Age at Menopause _____ yr

Dysmenorrhea: Present/absent   **Leucorrhea:** Present/absent   **Menorrhagia:** Present/absent

Marital History

Age at marriage _____ yrs   Duration of marriage _____ yrs

Consanguineous marriage—Yes/No   Relationship with spouse—satisfactory/unsatisfactory

Obstetric History

S. No	Year	Pregnancy (normal/ complicated)	Type of Delivery (Normal/Assisted/LSCS)	Place of Delivery (Hospital/ Home)	Delivery conducted by (Doctor/Nurse/ Dai/Other)	Alive/ Still borne	Sex	Birth- weight (in kg)	Present Condition (Alive/ dead)
1.									
2.									
3.									
4.									
5.									
6.									

Personal and Social History

Dietary pattern (veg/non-veg/lacto-ovo-vegetarian)/No. of meals per day/staple food/fasting habits

_____

_____

_____

_____

_____

Bowel and bladder habit (regular/irregular, stool frequency and consistency)

_____

_____

_____

_____

_____

Rest/sleep/activity/exercise/travel

_____

_____

_____

_____

Occupation (type/working hours per day/work place stress/job satisfaction)

_____

_____

_____

_____

_____

_____

Habits (alcohol/smoking/drugs/tobacco/chewing betel leaves)

_____

_____

_____

_____

_____

Leisure/recreational/religious/spiritual activities

_____

_____

_____

_____

_____

_____

Relationship with family members/relatives/friends/others—satisfactory/unsatisfactory

_____

_____

_____

_____

_____

_____

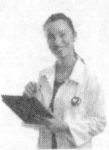

PHYSICAL EXAMINATION (put a tick (✓) mark wherever necessary or mention the finding in the provided space if needed)

General Appearance

Consciousness: Conscious/semi-conscious/unconscious/ confused
Posture: Normal/kyphosis/lordosis/scoliosis
Body built: Thin/moderate/obese
Nourishment: Well-nourished/under nourished
Activity: Active/dull/lethargic
Dress/grooming: Well-groomed/dirty
Gait (ability to walk/move): Normal/unsteady/any limp
Look: Normal/anxious/depressed/fear

Anthropometric Measurement

Weight: _____kg, Height: _____ cm, BMI (Quetelet's Index)_____[weight (kg)/height²(meter)]
Waist Circumference _____cm
 Hip Circumference _____cm
Waist/Hip Ratio- _____ (normal < 0.85)

Vital Signs

Temperature -_____°C, Pulse-_____beats/m,
Respiration _____breaths/m, BP _____ mm Hg,
Pain (5th vital sign)-absent/if present-onset/intensity/duration/ type/location
_____
_____
_____

Skin Condition

Color: Normal/redness/flushing/cyanosis/jaundice/ pallor/ pigmented/white patches
Texture: Smooth/soft/rough/dry/wrinkled/edematous
Lesions: Absent/macule/papule/vesicle/pustule/ulcer/scab
Temperature: Normal (warm)/cool/hot
Turgor (elasticity): Normal/decreased
_____

Head

Shape: Symmetrical/asymmetrical
Scalp: Normal/lesion/lump/infection/psoriasis
Hair: Colour: Normal/grey/white/artificial color
       Texture: Smooth/rough/dry/flaky/oily/thin
       Dandruff: Present/absent
       Alopecia: Present/absent
       Pediculosis: Present/absent
       Hygiene: Good/poor

Face

Shape: Symmetrical/asymmetrical
Color: Normal/pale/flushed
Edema: Present/absent
Movement: Normal/tics/tremors/fasciculation

Eyes

Eye	Right	Left
Discharge: Present/absent		
Eyebrows: Symmetrical/asymmetrical/absent		
Eyelids: Normal/edema/ptosis/entropion/ ectropion		
Eyelashes: Normal/stye/infection		
Eyeball: Normal/protruded/sunken		
Sclera: Normal/jaundice/redness		
Conjunctiva: Normal/moist/pale/red/watery/ purulent		
Pupils: Cloudy/dilated/constricted/reacting to light		
Vision: Normal/myopia/hyperopia		
Glasses/contact lens: Present/absent		

Ears

Ear	Right	Left
Shape: Symmetrical/asymmetrical with head		
External ear: Normal/discharge/earwax accumulation/pain/itching		
Auditory canal: Smooth/pink/redness/ discharge/wax plug/lesion/foreign body		
Tympanic membrane: Intact/redness/ swelling/perforated/bulging		
Gross Hearing: Normal/using hearing aid		

Nose

Discharge/crust: Present/absent
Nasal septum: Intact/perforated/deviation _____
Mucous membrane: Normal (moist & red)/dry/lesion/discharge/ swollen/epistaxis
Polyp: Present/absent
Flaring: Present/absent

Mouth

Odor: Normal/foul smelling
Lips: Normal (pink, moist, smooth)/dry/cracked/cyanosis/ swelling/redness/crust/cheilosis
Gums: Normal (pink and smooth)/swelling/bleeding/pus/ gingivitis
Tongue/mucus: Normal (pink and moist)/pale/dry/coated/ redness/lesion/swelling/glossitis
Teeth: Normal/poor alignment/missing/dental caries/plaque/ discoloration _____
Tonsils: Normal (small, pink, symmetrical)/inflammation/ enlarged/lesion/exudate
Throat and pharynx: Normal/redness/pus/lesion/exudate

contd…

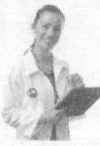

Neck

Lymph nodes (preauricular, parotid, postauricular, occipital, tonsillar, submaxillary, submental, anterior and deep cervical chain, posterior cervical, supraclavicular)- non-palpable/enlarge/tender

Thyroid gland: Normal (soft and elastic)/asymmetrical/enlarge/lump/bulging

Range of motion(flexion/extension/rotation): Symmetrical/asymmetrical neck with ROM

Chest

Shape/contour: Symmetrical/asymmetrical
Breathing pattern: Normal/unequal chest expansion/use of accessory muscles
Breath sounds: Normal/abnormal-wheezing/rhonchi/crackles/stridor/others _____
Sputum: Absent/if present, color/consistency _____
_____

Heart rate: Normal/fast/slow _____
Heart rhythm: Regular/irregular _____
Heart sounds: Normal/abnormal-murmur/others _____
_____

Female Breast

Breast	Right	Left
Size: Round/smooth/retraction/dimpling/lump/swollen/tender Shape: Symmetrical/asymmetrical _____		
Areola: Normal(moist, round)/dry Nipple: Everted/inversion/flat/cracked/crusted/discharge Axillary lymph nodes: Non-palpable/mobile/enlarge/tender Mass or lump: Absent/location/shape/size/consistency/tenderness _____		

Monthly Breast Self-Examination: Yes/No

Abdomen

Inspection
Shape: Symmetrical/asymmetrical/distension/observable mass/hernia/ascites/unusual pulsation
Color: Normal/white and silver lines (striae)
Skin: Normal/lesion/rashes/previous surgery scar/vascularity

Auscultation
Bowel sounds: Present/absent/frequency _____ movements/min

Palpation
Superficial palpation: Soft/pain/tenderness/mass _____
_____

Deep palpation (in all 4 quadrants for palpable organs): No organomegaly/pain/tenderness/palpable- liver/spleen/urinary bladder/appendix/inguinal hernia _____
Percussion: Presence of gas/fluid/mass (dullness)/liver margins
_____

Extremities

Upper extremities: Right Left	Right	Left
Range of motion: Symmetrical/asymmetrical		
Fingers: Normal/polydactyly/syndactyly arachnodactyly/edema/tremors/nodules/crepitus/pain		
Nails		
Color: Pink/pale/cyanosis		
Shape: Normal (convex)/spoon-shaped/beau's lines/flat/clubbed		
Hygiene: Clean/dirty/long/short		

Capillary refill time.......seconds (Normal<3 seconds)

Lower Extremities	Right	Left
Range of motion: Symmetrical/asymmetrical Toe/foot: Normal/polydactyly/syndactyly/arachnodactyly/nodule/edema/pain/alignment/position/shape _____		
Joint: Normal/warm/swollen/tender/painful		
Nails:		
Color: Pink/pale/cyanosis Shape: Normal (convex)/spoon-shaped/beau's lines/flat/clubbed Hygiene: Clean/dirty/long/short Varicose veins: Present/absent		

Rectum

Rectum and anus: Normal/hemorrhoids/fissures/polyp/ulcer/lesion/rashes/redness/bleeding
Stool: Color/odor/consistency _____
_____

Sacrococcygeal Area: Swelling/redness/dimpling or hair
Bowel pattern: Regular/irregular

Urinary Bladder

Bladder pattern: Normal/burning micturition/dribbling of urine while working or coughing
Urine: Color/odor/frequency _____

contd…

Genitals

Female Genitalia

Mons pubis: Normal/lesions/redness/edema
Labia majora: Normal/lesions/redness/edema
Perineum: Normal/lesions/redness/edema
Vagina: Normal/redness/lesion/discharge/pain _____
Urethra: Normal/discharge/redness/swelling _____
Inguinal lymph nodes: Normal/enlarge/tender/palpable

Male genitalia

Scrotum: Symmetrical/asymmetrical/lesions/redness/swelling/
pain/discharge/mass _____

_____

Penis: Normal/tenderness/pain/discharge
Foreskin: Intact/retractable/lesions
Location of urinary orifice: Normal/ventral/dorsal surface
Urethra: Normal/discharge/redness/swelling
Inguinal lymph nodes: Normal/enlarge/tender/palpable
Inguinal hernia: Absent/present
Monthly Testicular Self-Examination: Yes/No

LAB INVESTIGATIONS

S. No.	Date/time	Investigation	Patient value	Normal value	Remarks

MEDICATIONS

S. No.	Name and action	Dose/route/frequency	Indication	Side-effects

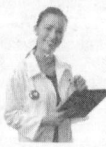

DIETARY PATTERN (24 HOURS RECALL)

Meal Time	Food item	Major Content	Quantity	Calories (kcal)	Carbohy-drate(g)	Protein (g)	Fat (g)	Iron (mg)	Calcium (mg)
Breakfast (__am)									
Midmorning (__am)									
Lunch (__pm)									
Evening Tea (__pm)									
Dinner (__pm)									
Bed time (__pm)									
Total									
Recommended Daily Values									
Deficient (–)/Excess (+)									

MODIFIED DIET PLAN

Meal Time	Food item	Major Content	Quantity	Calories (kcal)	Carbohy-drate(g)	Protein (g)	Fat (g)	Iron (mg)	Calcium (mg)
Breakfast (__am)									
Midmorning (__am)									
Lunch (__pm)									
Evening Tea (__pm)									
Dinner (__pm)									
Bed time (__pm)									
Total									
Recommended Daily Values									
Deficient (–)/Excess (+)									

Identified Health Problems/Needs

_____

_____

_____

_____

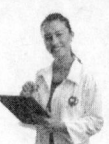

DISEASE CONDITION

(Book picture/comparison with available literature)

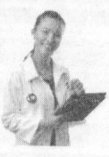

3. ELDERLY

Identification Data

Name: _____ Age/Sex _____

Classification/Diagnosis: _____

Brief History

History of present complaints (character/onset/location/duration/severity pattern/associated factors/medication and treatment)

_____

_____

_____

_____

_____

_____

_____

_____

_____

_____

_____

Past health (medical/surgical) history (problems at birth/infancy/childhood/immunization/adulthood (physical, mental, and psychological)/allergies (food/medication/others)/Chronic illness (e.g. hypertension, diabetes mellitus, heart, liver, renal disease etc./hereditary/communicable disease/any surgery and reason/other history)

_____

_____

_____

_____

_____

_____

_____

_____

_____

_____

_____

Menstrual History

Age at menarche: _____ yrs   **Menstruation:** Regular/irregular   **Length of cycle:** _____ days

Duration of blood flow: _____ days   **Dysmenorrhea:** Present/absent _____   **Leucorrhea:** Present/Absent _____

Menorrhagia: Present/absent   Age at Menopause_____ yr   **Postmenstrual bleeding:** Present/Absent ___

Marital History

Age at marriage _____ yrs   Duration of marriage _____ yrs   **Consanguineous marriage:** Yes/No

Relationship with spouse: Satisfactory/unsatisfactory   **Sexual activity:** Active/Inactive

Obstetric History

S. No	Year	Pregnancy (normal/ complicated)	Type of Delivery (Normal/Assisted/LSCS)	Place of Delivery (Hospital/ Home)	Delivery conducted by (Doctor/Nurse/ Dai/Other)	Alive/ still borne	Sex	Birth-weight (in kg)	Present Condition (Alive/ dead)
1.									
2.									
3.									
4.									
5.									
6.									

Personal and Social History

Dietary pattern (veg/non-veg/lacto-ovo-vegetarian)/No. of meals per day/staple food/fasting habits

_____

_____

_____

_____

Bowel and bladder habit (regular/irregular, stool frequency and consistency)

_____

_____

_____

_____

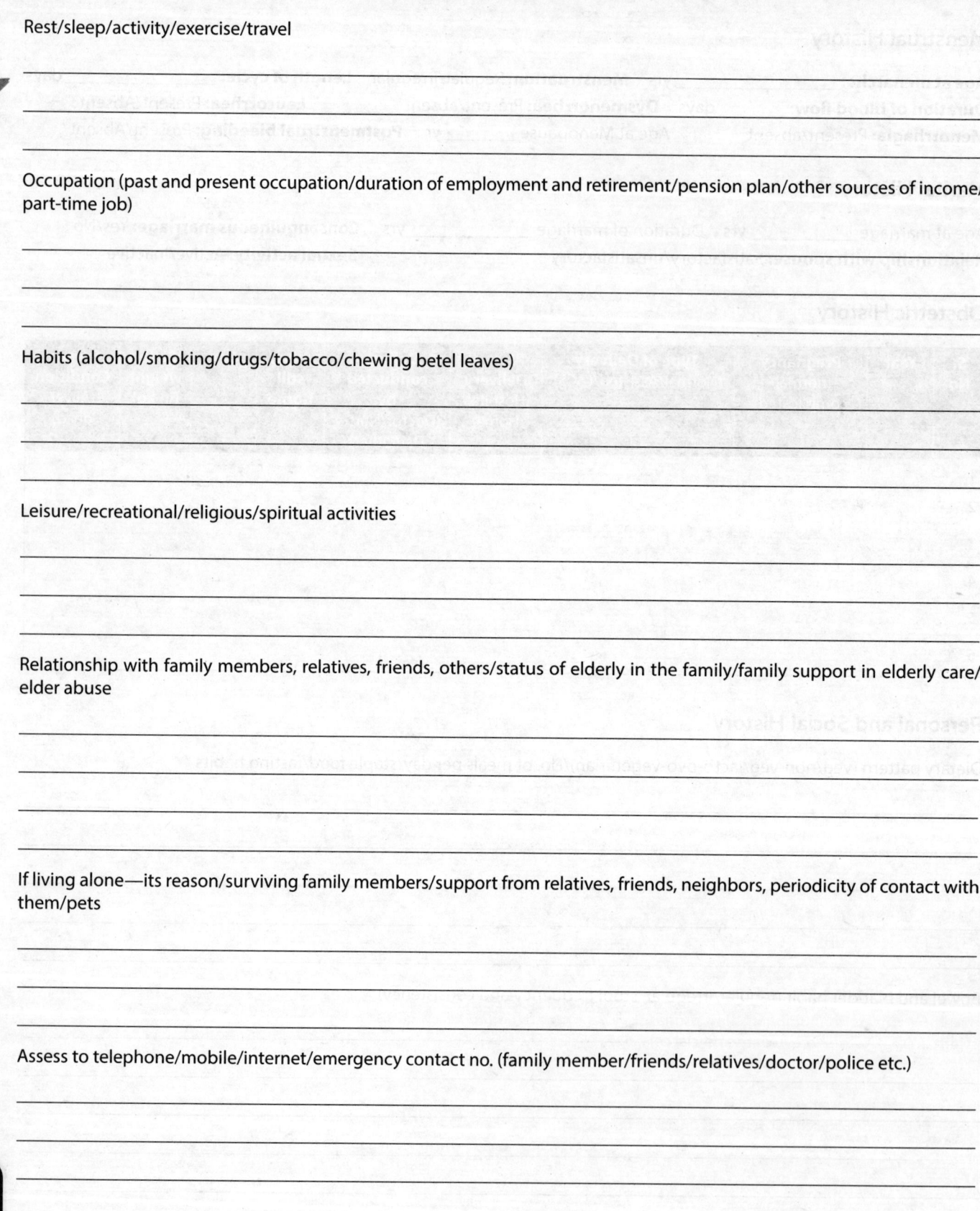

Rest/sleep/activity/exercise/travel

_____

_____

Occupation (past and present occupation/duration of employment and retirement/pension plan/other sources of income/part-time job)

_____

_____

_____

Habits (alcohol/smoking/drugs/tobacco/chewing betel leaves)

_____

_____

_____

Leisure/recreational/religious/spiritual activities

_____

_____

_____

Relationship with family members, relatives, friends, others/status of elderly in the family/family support in elderly care/elder abuse

_____

_____

_____

If living alone—its reason/surviving family members/support from relatives, friends, neighbors, periodicity of contact with them/pets

_____

_____

_____

Assess to telephone/mobile/internet/emergency contact no. (family member/friends/relatives/doctor/police etc.)

_____

_____

_____

_____

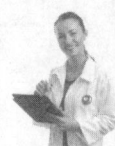

PHYSICAL EXAMINATION (put a tick (✓) mark wherever necessary or mention the finding in the provided space if needed)

General Appearance

Consciousness: Conscious/semi-conscious/unconscious/confused

Posture: Normal/kyphosis/lordosis/scoliosis

Body built: Thin/moderate/obese

Nourishment: Well-nourished/under nourished

Activity: Active/dull/lethargic

Dress/grooming: Well-groomed/dirty

Gait (ability to walk/move): Normal/unsteady/any limp

Look: Normal/anxious/depressed/fear

Anthropometric Measurement

Weight _____ kg, Height _____ cm, BMI (Quetelet's Index)_____ [weight (kg)/height²(meter)]

Waist Circumference _____ cm

Hip Circumference _____ cm

Waist/Hip Ratio- _____ (normal < 0.85)

Vital Signs

Temperature -_____°C, Pulse- _____beats/m,
Respiration _____ breaths/m, BP _____mm of Hg,
Pain (5th vital sign)-absent/if present-onset/intensity/duration/type/location

_____

_____

_____

Skin Condition

Color: Normal/pigmented/age spots/redness/flushing/cyanosis/jaundice/pallor/white patches

Texture: Smooth/soft/wrinkled/loose/scaling/sagging/rough/dry/oily/edematous

Eruptions: Absent/present _____

Itching: Absent/present _____

Masses: Absent/present _____

Unhealed or irregular sore/mole: Absent/present

Temperature: Normal (warm)/cool/hot

Bed sore: Present/absent

Head

Shape: Symmetrical/asymmetrical

Scalp: Normal/lesion/lump/infection/psoriasis

Hair: Colour: Normal/grey/white/artificial color

Texture: Smooth/rough/dry/flaky/oily/thin

Dandruff: Present/absent

Alopecia: Present/absent

Pediculosis: Present/absent

Hygiene: Good/poor

Face

Shape: Symmetrical/asymmetrical

Color: Normal/pale/flushed

Edema: Present/absent

Hirsutism: Present/absent

Eyes

Eye	Right	Left
Discharge: Present/absent		
Eyebrows: Symmetrical/asymmetrical/absent		
Eyelids: Normal/edema/ptosis/entropion/ectropion		
Eyelashes: Normal/stye/infection		
Eyeball: Normal/protruded/sunken		
Sclera: Normal/jaundice/redness		
Conjunctiva: Normal/moist/pale/red/watery/purulent		
Pupils: Cloudy/dilated/constricted/reacting to light		
Tearing: Present/absent		
Vision: Normal/myopia/hyperopia/blurred/glaucoma/cataract		
Glasses/contact lens: Present/absent		

Ears

Ear	Right	Left
External ear: Normal/discharge/earwax accumulation/pain/itching		
Auditory canal: Smooth/pink/redness/discharge/wax plug/lesion/foreign body		
Tympanic membrane: Intact/redness/swelling/perforated/bulging		
Gross hearing: Normal/difficulty in hearing/tinnitus/using hearing aid		

Nose

Discharge/crust: Present/absent

Nasal septum: Intact/perforated/deviation _____

Mucous membrane: Normal (moist & red)/dry/lesion/discharge/swollen/epistaxis

Polyp: Present/absent

Sense of smell: Normal decreased

Mouth

Odor: Normal/foul smelling

Lips: Normal (pink, moist, smooth)/dry/cracked/cyanosis/swelling/redness/crust/cheilosis

Gums: Normal (pink and smooth)/swelling/bleeding/pus/gingivitis

Tongue/mucus: Normal (pink and moist)/pale/dry/coated/fissures/redness/lesion/swelling/glossitis

45

contd...

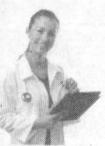

Teeth: Normal/missing/dentures/loose/dental caries/plaque/discoloration _____

Appetite: Normal/decreased

Sense of taste: Normal/altered

Chewing: Normal/difficult

Swallowing: Normal/difficult

Dry Mouth: Present/absent

Any devices: No/feeding tubes/parenteral nutrition/ostomy

Throat and pharynx: Normal/redness/pus/lesion/exudates

Monthly Oral Self-Examination: yes/no

Neck

Lymph nodes (preauricular, parotid, postauricular, occipital, tonsillar, submaxillary, submental, anterior and deep cervical chain, posterior cervical, supraclavicular)- non-palpable/enlarge/tender

Thyroid gland: Normal (soft and elastic)/asymmetrical/enlarge/lump/bulging

Neck movement: Normal/pain/stiffness

Chest

Shape/contour: Symmetrical/asymmetrical

Breathing pattern: Normal/dyspnea/excessive sneezing/excessive coughing/unequal chest expansion/pain in exertion/palpitation in exertion/shortness of breath

Breath sounds: Normal/abnormal-wheezing/rhonchi/crackles/stridor/others _____

Sputum: Absent/if present, color/consistency _____

Heart rate: Normal/fast/slow _____

Heart rhythm: Regular/irregular _____

Heart sounds: Normal/abnormal-murmur/others _____

Blood Pressure: Normal/decreased/increased

Exercise intolerance: Present/absent

Female Breast

Breast	Right	Left
Size: Round/pendulous/retraction/dimpling/lump/tender		
Shape: Symmetrical/asymmetrical		
Areola: Normal(moist, round)/dry		
Nipple: Normal/everted/inversion/flat/cracked/crusted/any discharge		
Axillary lymph nodes: Non-palpable/mobile/enlarge/tender		
Mass or lump: Absent/if present, location/shape/size/consistency/tenderness		

Monthly Breast Self-Examination: Yes/No

Abdomen

Inspection

Shape: Symmetrical/asymmetrical/distension/observable mass/hernia/ascites/unusual pulsation

Color: Normal/white and silver lines (striae)

Skin: Normal/lesion/rashes/previous surgery scar/vascularity

Auscultation

Bowel sounds: Present/absent/frequency ___ movements/min

Palpation

Superficial palpation: Soft/pain/tenderness/mass _____

Deep palpation (in all 4 quadrants for palpable organs) – no organomegaly/pain/tenderness/palpable- liver/spleen/urinary bladder/appendix/inguinal hernia _____

Percussion: Presence of gas/fluid/mass (dullness)/liver margins _____

Digestion: Normal/sluggish/heart burn/belching/distension

Extremities

Upper extremities	Right	Left
Range of motion: Symmetrical/asymmetrical/decreased		
Fingers: Normal/polydactylyl/syndactyl/rachnodactyl/edema/tremors (shaking)/nodules/crepitus/pain		
Joint: Normal/stiffness/warm/swollen/tender/painful		
Nails: Color-pink/pale/cyanosis		
Shape/texture: Normal (convex)/spoon-shaped/beau's lines/flat/clubbed/thick/brittle		
Nail hygiene: Clean/dirty/long/short		

Capillary refill time _____ seconds (Normal<3 seconds)

Lower extremities	Right	Left
Range of motion-symmetrical/asymmetrical/decreased		
Toe/foot: Normal/polydactyly/syndactyly/arachnodactyly/nodule/edema/pain/alignment/position/shape _____		
Joint: Normal/stiffness/warm/swollen /tender/painful		
Nails: Color-pink/pale/cyanosis		
Shape/texture: Normal (convex)/spoon-shaped/beau's lines/flat/clubbed/thick/brittle		
Use of walking aid: No/If yes—stick/crutches/prosthesis		
Hygiene: Clean/dirty/long/short		
Varicose veins: Present/absent		

Rectum

Rectum and anus: Normal/hemorrhoids/fissures/polyp/ulcer/lesion/rashes/redness/bleeding

Stool: Color/odor/consistency _____

Bowel pattern: Regular/irregular

Defecation: Normal/painful/bleeding/diarrhea/constipation

contd…

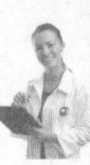

Urinary Bladder

Bladder pattern: Normal/dysuria/nocturia/hematuria/polyuria/burning micturition/dribbling of urine while working or coughing/incontinence

Urine: Color/odor/frequency _____

_____

Genitals

Female Genitalia

Vagina: Normal/itching/dry/pain/redness/lesion/discharge

Urethra: Normal/discharge/redness/swelling _____

Inguinal lymph nodes: Normal/enlarge/tender/palpable

Male Genitalia

Scrotum: Normal/pendulous/symmetrical/asymmetrical/lesions/redness/swelling/pain/discharge/mass _____

Penis: Normal/tenderness/pain/discharge/lesions

Urethra: Normal/discharge/redness/swelling

Inguinal lymph nodes: Normal/enlarge/tender/palpable

Inguinal hernia: Absent/present

Monthly Testicular Self-Examination: Yes/No

Neurological Assessment

Coordination and balance: Normal/decrease/abnormal

Pain perception: Normal/decrease/absent

Touch perception: Normal/decrease/absent

Hot perception: Normal/decrease/absent

Cold perception: Normal/decrease/absent

Headache/seizures: Absent/present

Syncope/fainting attacks: Absent/present

Dizziness: Absent/present

Giddiness: Absent/present

Numbness in hand or feet: Absent/present

Tremors: Absent/present

Dementia/Forgetfulness

Recall 3 items at 1 minute: <2 items/2 items/all 3 items

Name as many as animals as in 1 minutes: Normal (able to recall 18 or more animals in 1 minute)/abnormal (able to recall less than 12 animals in 1 minute)

ACTIVITIES OF DAILY LIVING (ADL)

S. No.	Daily living activities	Yes/No
	Personal tasks	
1.	Eat food by self	
2.	Drink fluids by self	
3.	Go to toilet by self	
4.	Able to control bladder	
5.	Able to control bowel	
6.	Go to bathroom by self	
7.	Bath by self	
8.	Dress and undress by self	
9.	Cut or clean nails by self	
10.	Comb and tie hairs by self	
11.	Able to move independently	
12.	Able to sit down in chair/bed by self	
13.	Able to climb stairs	
	Household Tasks	
14.	Perform routine household work (e.g. bed making, arranging furniture)	
15.	Wash clothes	
16.	Cooking	

contd...

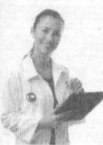

S. No.	Daily living activities	Yes/No
17.	Keep living place clean and tidy	
18.	Open or close doors and windows of living room	
19.	Go to the market	
20.	Manage finances	
21.	Gardening	
	Outside Tasks	
22.	Meaningful leisure time activities (e.g. reading newspapers, social/religious gathering)	
23.	Go for an outing	
24.	Verbally communicate with relatives and friends	
25.	Communicate in writing (e.g. writing letters) with relatives/friends	
26.	Go to the temple/religious places	
27.	Go to a long distance for shopping	
28.	Go to the doctor/clinic	
29.	Go to the bank	
30.	Go do full time/part time job	

RISK OF ACCIDENT/INJURIES IN SURROUNDING ENVIRONMENT

S. No.	Risk of accident/injuries	Yes/No
1.	Slippery floor	
2.	Stagnant water on floor/bathroom	
3.	Inadequate lighting in passages/stairs/living room/bathroom	
4.	Furniture/objects in the passages or corridors	
5.	High height beds/Bed without side rails	
6.	High heeled/loose fitting shoes/slippers	
7.	No hearing aid with poor hearing acuity/Non-working hearing aid	
8.	No spectacles with blurred vision/Wearing new spectacles	
9.	Inability to recognize the temperature of water before bath/drink/hot water bottles	
10.	Keeping the medications or drinks unlabeled/near to the poisonous substances	

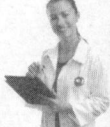

LAB INVESTIGATIONS

S. No.	Date/time	Investigation	Patient value	Normal value	Remarks

MEDICATIONS

S. No.	Name and action	Dose/route/frequency	Indication	Side-effects

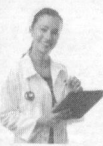

DIETARY PATTERN (24 HOURS RECALL)

Meal Time	Food item	Major Content	Quantity	Calories (kcal)	Carbohy-drate(g)	Protein (g)	Fat (g)	Iron (mg)	Calcium (mg)
Breakfast (__am)									
Midmorning (__am)									
Lunch (__pm)									
Evening Tea (__pm)									
Dinner (__pm)									
Bed time (__pm)									
Total									
Recommended Daily Values									
Deficient (–)/Excess (+)									

MODIFIED DIET PLAN

Meal Time	Food item	Major Content	Quantity	Calories (kcal)	Carbohy-drate(g)	Protein (g)	Fat (g)	Iron (mg)	Calcium (mg)
Breakfast (__am)									
Midmorning (__am)									
Lunch (__pm)									
Evening Tea (__pm)									
Dinner (__pm)									
Bed time (__pm)									
Total									
Recommended Daily Values									
Deficient (–)/Excess (+)									

Identified Health Problems/Needs

_____

_____

_____

_____

DISEASE CONDITION

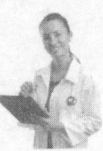

(Book picture/comparison with available literature)

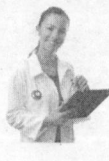

4. ELDERLY

Identification Data

Name: _____ Age/Sex _____
Classification/Diagnosis: _____

Brief History

History of present complaints (character/onset/location/duration/severity pattern/associated factors/medication and treatment)

_____
_____
_____
_____
_____
_____
_____
_____
_____
_____

Past health (medical/surgical) history (problems at birth/infancy/childhood/immunization/adulthood (physical, mental, and psychological)/allergies (food/medication/others)/Chronic illness (e.g. hypertension, diabetes mellitus, heart, liver, renal disease etc./hereditary/communicable disease/any surgery and reason/other history)

_____
_____
_____
_____
_____
_____
_____
_____
_____
_____

Menstrual History

Age at menarche: _____ yrs   **Menstruation:** Regular/irregular   **Length of cycle:** _____ days
Duration of blood flow: _____ days   **Dysmenorrhea:** Present/absent _____   **Leucorrhea:** Present/Absent ____
Menorrhagia: Present/absent   Age at Menopause_____ yr   **Postmenstrual bleeding:** Present/Absent ___

Marital History

Age at marriage _____ yrs   Duration of marriage _____ yrs   **Consanguineous marriage:** Yes/No
Relationship with spouse: Satisfactory/unsatisfactory   **Sexual activity:** Active/Inactive

Obstetric History

S. No	Year	Pregnancy (normal/ complicated)	Type of Delivery (Normal/Assisted/LSCS)	Place of Delivery (Hospital/ Home)	Delivery conducted by (Doctor/Nurse/ Dai/Other)	Alive/ still borne	Sex	Birth- weight (in kg)	Present Condition (Alive/ dead)
1.									
2.									
3.									
4.									
5.									
6.									

Personal and Social History

Dietary pattern (veg/non-veg/lacto-ovo-vegetarian)/No. of meals per day/staple food/fasting habits

_____

_____

_____

_____

Bowel and bladder habit (regular/irregular, stool frequency and consistency)

_____

_____

_____

_____

_____

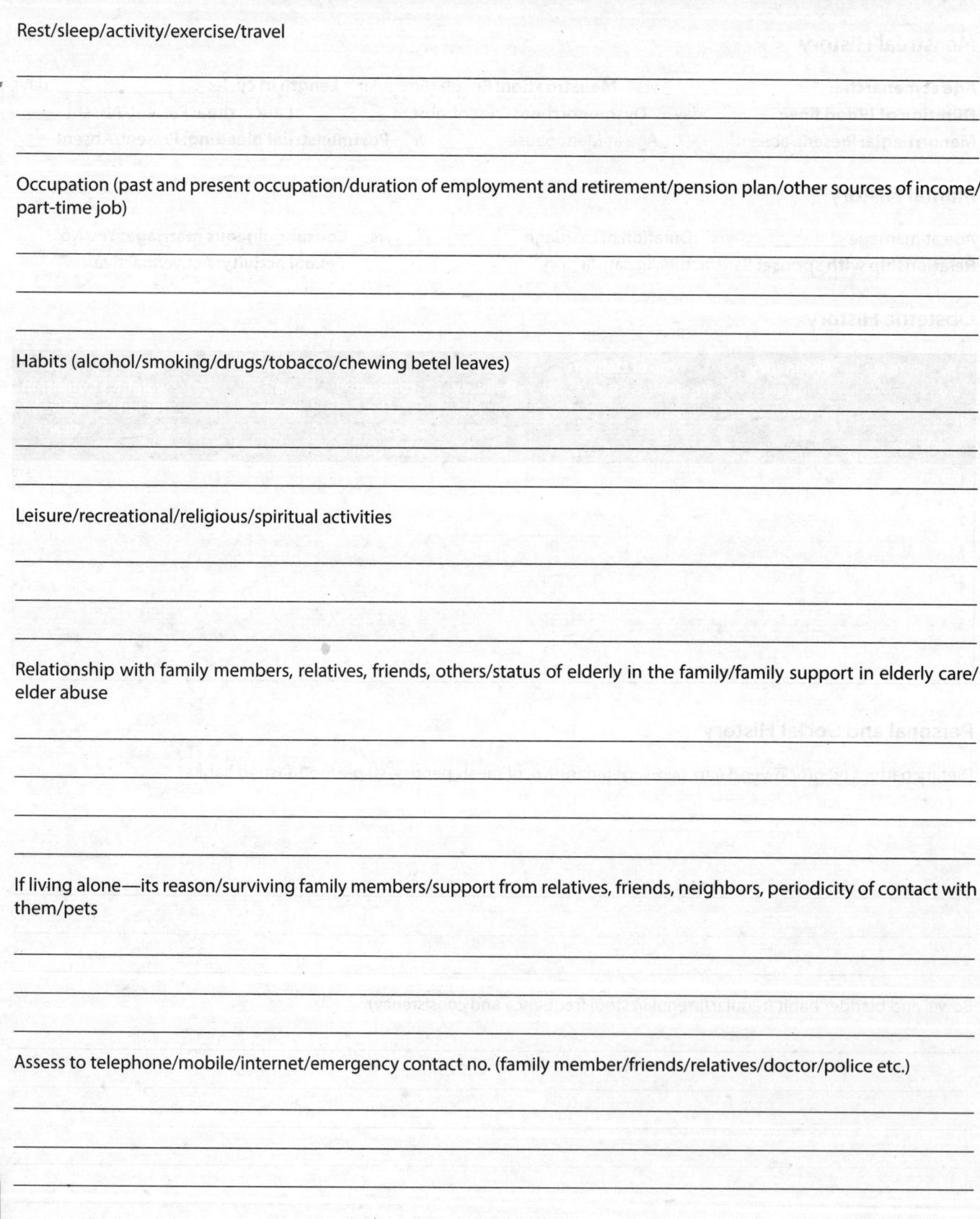

Rest/sleep/activity/exercise/travel

_____

_____

_____

Occupation (past and present occupation/duration of employment and retirement/pension plan/other sources of income/part-time job)

_____

_____

_____

Habits (alcohol/smoking/drugs/tobacco/chewing betel leaves)

_____

_____

_____

_____

Leisure/recreational/religious/spiritual activities

_____

_____

_____

_____

Relationship with family members, relatives, friends, others/status of elderly in the family/family support in elderly care/elder abuse

_____

_____

_____

_____

If living alone—its reason/surviving family members/support from relatives, friends, neighbors, periodicity of contact with them/pets

_____

_____

_____

Assess to telephone/mobile/internet/emergency contact no. (family member/friends/relatives/doctor/police etc.)

_____

_____

_____

_____

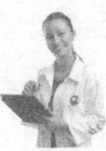

PHYSICAL EXAMINATION (put a tick (✓) mark wherever necessary or mention the finding in the provided space if needed)

General Appearance

Consciousness: Conscious/semi-conscious/unconscious/confused
Posture: Normal/kyphosis/lordosis/scoliosis
Body built: Thin/moderate/obese
Nourishment: Well-nourished/under nourished
Activity: Active/dull/lethargic
Dress/grooming: Well-groomed/dirty
Gait (ability to walk/move): Normal/unsteady/any limp
Look: Normal/anxious/depressed/fear

Anthropometric Measurement

Weight _____ kg, Height _____ cm, BMI (Quetelet's Index) _____ [weight (kg)/height^2(meter)]
Waist Circumference _____ cm
Hip Circumference _____ cm
Waist/Hip Ratio- _____ (normal < 0.85)

Vital Signs

Temperature - _____ °C, Pulse- _____ beats/m,
Respiration _____ breaths/m, BP _____ mm of Hg,
Pain (5th vital sign)-absent/if present-onset/intensity/duration/type/location

_____

_____

_____

Skin Condition

Color: Normal/pigmented/age spots/redness/flushing/cyanosis/jaundice/pallor/white patches
Texture: Smooth/soft/wrinkled/loose/scaling/sagging/rough/dry/oily/edematous
Eruptions: Absent/present _____
Itching: Absent/present _____
Masses: Absent/present _____
Unhealed or irregular sore/mole: Absent/present
Temperature: Normal (warm)/cool/hot
Bed sore: Present/absent

Head

Shape: Symmetrical/asymmetrical
Scalp: Normal/lesion/lump/infection/psoriasis
Hair: Colour: Normal/grey/white/artificial color
  Texture: Smooth/rough/dry/flaky/oily/thin
  Dandruff: Present/absent
  Alopecia: Present/absent
  Pediculosis: Present/absent
  Hygiene: Good/poor

Face

Shape: Symmetrical/asymmetrical
Color: Normal/pale/flushed

Edema: Present/absent
Hirsutism: Present/absent

Eyes

Eye	Right	Left
Discharge: Present/absent		
Eyebrows: Symmetrical/asymmetrical/absent		
Eyelids: Normal/edema/ptosis/entropion/ectropion		
Eyelashes: Normal/stye/infection		
Eyeball: Normal/protruded/sunken		
Sclera: Normal/jaundice/redness		
Conjunctiva: Normal/moist/pale/red/watery/purulent		
Pupils: Cloudy/dilated/constricted/reacting to light		
Tearing: Present/absent		
Vision: Normal/myopia/hyperopia/blurred/glaucoma/cataract		
Glasses/contact lens: Present/absent		

Ears

Ear	Right	Left
External ear: Normal/discharge/earwax accumulation/pain/itching		
Auditory canal: Smooth/pink/redness/discharge/wax plug/lesion/foreign body		
Tympanic membrane: Intact/redness/swelling/perforated/bulging		
Gross hearing: Normal/difficulty in hearing/tinnitus/using hearing aid		

Nose

Discharge/crust: Present/absent
Nasal septum: Intact/perforated/deviation _____
Mucous membrane: Normal (moist & red)/dry/lesion/discharge/swollen/epistaxis
Polyp: Present/absent
Sense of smell: Normal decreased

Mouth

Odor: Normal/foul smelling
Lips: Normal (pink, moist, smooth)/dry/cracked/cyanosis/swelling/redness/crust/cheilosis
Gums: Normal (pink and smooth)/swelling/bleeding/pus/gingivitis
Tongue/mucus: Normal (pink and moist)/pale/dry/coated/fissures/redness/lesion/swelling/glossitis

55

contd…

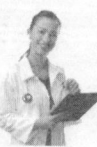

Teeth: Normal/missing/dentures/loose/dental caries/plaque/discoloration _____

Appetite: Normal/decreased

Sense of taste: Normal/altered

Chewing: Normal/difficult

Swallowing: Normal/difficult

Dry Mouth: Present/absent

Any devices: No/feeding tubes/parenteral nutrition/ostomy

Throat and pharynx: Normal/redness/pus/lesion/exudates

Monthly Oral Self-Examination: yes/no

Neck

Lymph nodes (preauricular, parotid, postauricular, occipital, tonsillar, submaxillary, submental, anterior and deep cervical chain, posterior cervical, supraclavicular)- non-palpable/enlarge/tender

Thyroid gland: Normal (soft and elastic)/asymmetrical/enlarge/lump/bulging

Neck movement: Normal/pain/stiffness

Chest

Shape/contour: Symmetrical/asymmetrical

Breathing pattern: Normal/dyspnea/excessive sneezing/excessive coughing/unequal chest expansion/pain in exertion/palpitation in exertion/shortness of breath

Breath sounds: Normal/abnormal-wheezing/rhonchi/crackles/stridor/others _____

Sputum: Absent/if present, color/consistency _____

_____

Heart rate: Normal/fast/slow _____

Heart rhythm: Regular/irregular _____

Heart sounds: Normal/abnormal-murmur/others _____

Blood Pressure: Normal/decreased/increased

Exercise intolerance: Present/absent

Female Breast

Breast	Right	Left
Size: Round/pendulous/retraction/dimpling/lump/tender		
Shape: Symmetrical/asymmetrical		
Areola: Normal(moist, round)/dry		
Nipple: Normal/everted/inversion/flat/cracked/crusted/any discharge		
Axillary lymph nodes: Non-palpable/mobile/enlarge/tender		
Mass or lump: Absent/if present, location/shape/size/consistency/tenderness		

Monthly Breast Self-Examination: Yes/No

Abdomen

Inspection

Shape: Symmetrical/asymmetrical/distension/observable mass/hernia/ascites/unusual pulsation

Color: Normal/white and silver lines (striae)

Skin: Normal/lesion/rashes/previous surgery scar/vascularity

Auscultation

Bowel sounds: Present/absent/frequency ___ movements/min

Palpation

Superficial palpation: Soft/pain/tenderness/mass _____

_____

Deep palpation (in all 4 quadrants for palpable organs) – no organomegaly/pain/tenderness/palpable- liver/spleen/urinary bladder/appendix/inguinal hernia _____

Percussion: Presence of gas/fluid/mass (dullness)/liver margins

_____

Digestion: Normal/sluggish/heart burn/belching/distension

Extremities

Upper extremities	Right	Left
Range of motion: Symmetrical/asymmetrical/decreased		
Fingers: Normal/polydactylyl/syndactyl/rachnodactyl/edema/tremors (shaking)/nodules/crepitus/pain		
Joint: Normal/stiffness/warm/swollen/tender/painful		
Nails: Color-pink/pale/cyanosis		
Shape/texture: Normal (convex)/spoon-shaped/beau's lines/flat/clubbed/thick/brittle		
Nail hygiene: Clean/dirty/long/short		

Capillary refill time _____ seconds (Normal<3 seconds)

Lower extremities	Right	Left
Range of motion-symmetrical/asymmetrical/decreased		
Toe/foot: Normal/polydactyly/syndactyly/arachnodactyly/nodule/edema/pain/alignment/position/shape _____		
Joint: Normal/stiffness/warm/swollen /tender/painful		
Nails: Color-pink/pale/cyanosis		
Shape/texture: Normal (convex)/spoon-shaped/beau's lines/flat/clubbed/thick/brittle		
Use of walking aid: No/If yes—stick/crutches/prosthesis		
Hygiene: Clean/dirty/long/short		
Varicose veins: Present/absent		

Rectum

Rectum and anus: Normal/hemorrhoids/fissures/polyp/ulcer/lesion/rashes/redness/bleeding

Stool: Color/odor/consistency _____

_____

Bowel pattern: Regular/irregular

Defecation: Normal/painful/bleeding/diarrhea/constipation

contd...

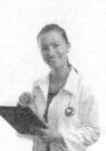

Urinary Bladder

Bladder pattern: Normal/dysuria/nocturia/hematuria/polyuria/
burning micturition/dribbling of urine while working or
coughing/incontinence
Urine: Color/odor/frequency _____
_____

Genitals

Female Genitalia

Vagina: Normal/itching/dry/pain/redness/lesion/discharge
Urethra: Normal/discharge/redness/swelling _____
Inguinal lymph nodes: Normal/enlarge/tender/palpable

Male Genitalia

Scrotum: Normal/pendulous/symmetrical/asymmetrical/lesions/
redness/swelling/pain/discharge/mass _____
Penis: Normal/tenderness/pain/discharge/lesions
Urethra: Normal/discharge/redness/swelling
Inguinal lymph nodes: Normal/enlarge/tender/palpable
Inguinal hernia: Absent/present
Monthly Testicular Self-Examination: Yes/No

Neurological Assessment

Coordination and balance: Normal/decrease/abnormal
Pain perception: Normal/decrease/absent
Touch perception: Normal/decrease/absent
Hot perception: Normal/decrease/absent
Cold perception: Normal/decrease/absent
Headache/seizures: Absent/present
Syncope/fainting attacks: Absent/present
Dizziness: Absent/present
Giddiness: Absent/present
Numbness in hand or feet: Absent/present
Tremors: Absent/present

Dementia/Forgetfulness

Recall 3 items at 1 minute: <2 items/2 items/all 3 items
Name as many as animals as in 1 minutes: Normal (able to recall
18 or more animals in 1 minute)/abnormal (able to recall less
than 12 animals in 1 minute)

ACTIVITIES OF DAILY LIVING (ADL)

S. No.	Daily living activities	Yes/No
	Personal tasks	
1.	Eat food by self	
2.	Drink fluids by self	
3.	Go to toilet by self	
4.	Able to control bladder	
5.	Able to control bowel	
6.	Go to bathroom by self	
7.	Bath by self	
8.	Dress and undress by self	
9.	Cut or clean nails by self	
10.	Comb and tie hairs by self	
11.	Able to move independently	
12.	Able to sit down in chair/bed by self	
13.	Able to climb stairs	
	Household Tasks	
14.	Perform routine household work (e.g. bed making, arranging furniture)	
15.	Wash clothes	
16.	Cooking	

contd…

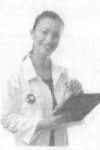

S. No.	Daily living activities	Yes/No
17.	Keep living place clean and tidy	
18.	Open or close doors and windows of living room	
19.	Go to the market	
20.	Manage finances	
21.	Gardening	
	Outside Tasks	
22.	Meaningful leisure time activities (e.g. reading newspapers, social/religious gathering)	
23.	Go for an outing	
24.	Verbally communicate with relatives and friends	
25.	Communicate in writing (e.g. writing letters) with relatives/friends	
26.	Go to the temple/religious places	
27.	Go to a long distance for shopping	
28.	Go to the doctor/clinic	
29.	Go to the bank	
30.	Go do full time/part time job	

RISK OF ACCIDENT/INJURIES IN SURROUNDING ENVIRONMENT

S. No.	Risk of accident/injuries	Yes/No
1.	Slippery floor	
2.	Stagnant water on floor/bathroom	
3.	Inadequate lighting in passages/stairs/living room/bathroom	
4.	Furniture/objects in the passages or corridors	
5.	High height beds/Bed without side rails	
6.	High heeled/loose fitting shoes/slippers	
7.	No hearing aid with poor hearing acuity/Non-working hearing aid	
8.	No spectacles with blurred vision/Wearing new spectacles	
9.	Inability to recognize the temperature of water before bath/drink/hot water bottles	
10.	Keeping the medications or drinks unlabeled/near to the poisonous substances	

LAB INVESTIGATIONS

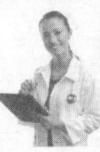

S. No.	Date/time	Investigation	Patient value	Normal value	Remarks

MEDICATIONS

S. No.	Name and action	Dose/route/frequency	Indication	Side-effects

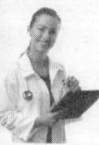

DIETARY PATTERN (24 HOURS RECALL)

Meal Time	Food item	Major Content	Quantity	Calories (kcal)	Carbohy-drate(g)	Protein (g)	Fat (g)	Iron (mg)	Calcium (mg)
Breakfast (__am)									
Midmorning (__am)									
Lunch (__pm)									
Evening Tea (__pm)									
Dinner (__pm)									
Bed time (__pm)									
Total									
Recommended Daily Values									
Deficient (–)/Excess (+)									

MODIFIED DIET PLAN

Meal Time	Food item	Major Content	Quantity	Calories (kcal)	Carbohy-drate(g)	Protein (g)	Fat (g)	Iron (mg)	Calcium (mg)
Breakfast (__am)									
Midmorning (__am)									
Lunch (__pm)									
Evening Tea (__pm)									
Dinner (__pm)									
Bed time (__pm)									
Total									
Recommended Daily Values									
Deficient (–)/Excess (+)									

Identified Health Problems/Needs

_____

_____

_____

_____

DISEASE CONDITION

(Book picture/comparison with available literature)

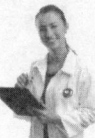

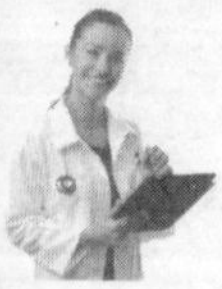

OTHERS FAMILY MEMBERS

5. _____

_____

_____

_____

_____

_____

_____

_____

_____

_____

_____

_____

_____

_____

_____

_____

_____

_____

_____

_____

_____

_____

_____

_____

_____

_____

_____

_____

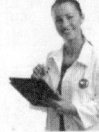

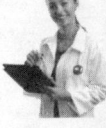

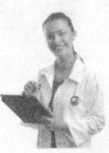

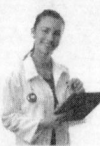

Instructions

1. Write the family health nursing care plan for at least 3 consecutive days.
2. For each day, identify the family health needs, prioritize them and formulate the possible nursing diagnosis.
3. If more details are required, paste the additional pages in the record book.

IDENTIFIED HEALTH PROBLEMS/NEEDS

DAY-1   Date-

_____

_____

_____

_____

DAY-2   Date-

_____

_____

_____

DAY-3   Date-

_____

_____

_____

Prioritization of Health Problems/Needs

DAY-1

_____

_____

_____

_____

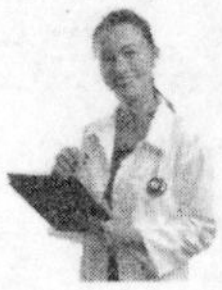

DAY-2

_____

_____

_____

_____

DAY-3

_____

_____

_____

_____

Priority Nursing Diagnosis

DAY-1

_____

_____

_____

_____

DAY-2

_____

_____

_____

_____

DAY-3

_____

_____

_____

_____

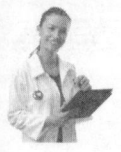

FAMILY HEALTH NURSING CARE PLAN (DAY-1)

DATE-

Assessment	Diagnosis	Goal/ Objective	Planning	Implementation	Evaluation

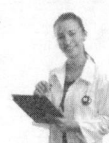

FAMILY HEALTH NURSING CARE PLAN (DAY-1)

Assessment	Diagnosis	Goal/ Objective	Planning	Implementation	Evaluation

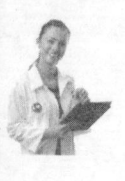

FAMILY HEALTH NURSING CARE PLAN (DAY-1)

Assessment	Diagnosis	Goal/ Objective	Planning	Implementation	Evaluation

HEALTH EDUCATION

DATE-

FAMILY HEALTH NURSING CARE PLAN (DAY-2)

Assessment	Diagnosis	Goal/ Objective	Planning	Implementation	Evaluation

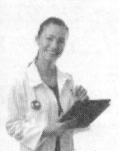

FAMILY HEALTH NURSING CARE PLAN (DAY-2)

Assessment	Diagnosis	Goal/ Objective	Planning	Implementation	Evaluation

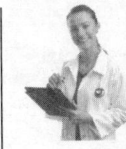

FAMILY HEALTH NURSING CARE PLAN (DAY-2)

Assessment	Diagnosis	Goal/ Objective	Planning	Implementation	Evaluation

HEALTH EDUCATION

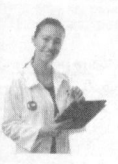

FAMILY HEALTH NURSING CARE PLAN (DAY-3)

DATE-

Assessment	Diagnosis	Goal/ Objective	Planning	Implementation	Evaluation

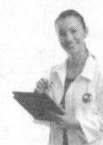

FAMILY HEALTH NURSING CARE PLAN (DAY-3)

Assessment	Diagnosis	Goal/ Objective	Planning	Implementation	Evaluation

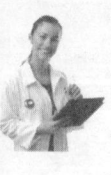

FAMILY HEALTH NURSING CARE PLAN (DAY-3)

Assessment	Diagnosis	Goal/ Objective	Planning	Implementation	Evaluation

HEALTH EDUCATION

REFERENCES

Signature of Student

Signature of Supervisor

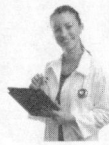

3. Family Health Nursing Care Plan

IDENTIFICATION DATA

Name of the Area: _____

Name of Informant: _____

Relationship with Head of Family: _____

Age/Sex: _____

House No.: _____

Date of Starting: _____

Date of Ending: _____

INTRODUCTION OF THE FAMILY

General Information

Name of Head of the Family: _____

Address: _____

Religion—Hindu/Muslims/Sikh/Christian/Others: _____

Caste—GEN/SC/ST/OBC: _____

Occupation of the head of the family: Unemployed/Government/Private Job/Self-Employed/Daily Wage Worker/ Homemaker/Others: _____

Language known: Hindi/English/Others: _____

Family Size (Total Members): _____

Family Type: Nuclear/Joint: _____

Ownership of House: Own/Rented: _____

Monthly Family Income: ₹: _____

Family Income per Capita: ₹: _____

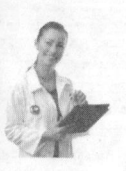

FAMILY COMPOSITION AND CHARACTERISTICS

S. No.	Name of the family members	Relationship with head of the family	Date of birth/sex (Male-M/Female-F/ Transgender-T)	Marital status (Unmarried/ married)	Educational status	Occupation	Monthly income (₹)	Dietary habits (veg/non-veg)	Addiction (smoking alcohol/ drugs/ others)	Health status (healthy/ unhealthy)
1.										
2.										
3.										
4.										
5.										
6.										
7.										
8.										

Key

Family Tree/Genogramme

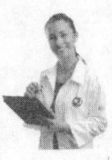

AVAILABILITY OF HEALTH CARE/SOCIAL/EDUCATIONAL FACILITIES

Facilities	Yes/No (If yes, specify name and distance from the house)
Nearby Health care facilities	
District hospital	
Government maternity hospital (if any)	
Private hospitals	
Sub center	
Primary health center	
Community health center	
Indigenous medicine (hospital/clinic/dispensary)	
• Ayurveda	
• Yoga	
• Naturopathy	
• Unani	
• Siddha	
• Homeopathy	
• If other, specify	
Non-Governmental Organizations/Voluntary Health Organizations	
• Orphan age children	
• Physically challenged	
• Visually challenged	
• Mentally challenged	
• Hearing challenged	
• Women	
• Elderly	
• Youth welfare	
• Other	
Social Agencies	
• Post office	
• Bank	
• Police station	
Education facilities	
Government	
• Anganwadis	
• Balwadis	
• Primary school	
• Elementary school	
• Secondary school	
• Senior secondary school	
• UG Institutions	
• PG institutions	
Private	
• Primary school	
• Elementary school	
• Secondary school	
• Senior secondary school	
• UG Institutions	
• PG institutions	

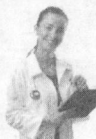

AVAILABILITY OF RECREATION/COMMUNICATION/TRANSPORT/RELIGIOUS FACILITIES

Facilities	Yes/No (If yes, specify name and distance from the house)
Recreation facilities	
• Nearby market	
• Playgrounds	
• Public Gardens	
• Cinema halls	
• Clubs	
• Public Library	
• Fairs	
• Festivals	
Communication facilities	
• Telephone connection	
• Mobile phone	
• Internet facility	
• Letters	
Transport facilities	
• Bus	
• Auto rickshaw	
• Taxi	
• Four wheeler	
• Two wheeler	
• Train	
• Airway	
Religious places	
• Temple	
• Mosque	
• Gurudwara	
• Church	

Sketch of House

(Draw a sketch of the house showing location of rooms, doors, windows, entrance of the house, drinking water source, toilet, kitchen)

HOUSING STANDARDS AND ENVIRONMENTAL CONDITIONS

Characteristic	Parameters
Type of house	Pucca/Semi pucca/Katcha
Site	Elevated from surroundings/depressed from surroundings
Total number of living room	1/2/3/4/5/6/7/8/ _____
Space per person	Adequate (1 room -2 persons, 2 rooms -3 persons, 3 rooms – 5 persons, 4 rooms -7 persons, 5 or more rooms - 10 persons (additional 2 for each further room Inadequate (if above criteria is not fulfilled)
Ventilation	Adequate (doors and windows facing each other in each room) Inadequate (doors and windows not facing each other in each room)
Bathroom Hygiene	Not available/If available—Own/Public Hygienic/Unhygienic
Wall	Plastered or Cemented/Tiled/Wooden/Unplastered/Mud//Others, specify _____

Roof
  Height
  Painting
	
	Less than 10 feet/More than 10 feet
	Light colored/Dark colored

Day light	Adequate (Able to read the small fonts of newspaper inside the room during the day without any artificial lighting) Inadequate (Not able to read the small fonts of newspaper inside the room during the day without any artificial lighting)
Latrine Hygiene	Not available/If available—Own/Public Hygienic/Unhygienic
Electricity	Not available/Available
Drinking water supply	Tap/Well/Lake/Pond/Others, specify _____
Kitchen	Separate/Corner of the room/Others, specify _____
Type of fuel used	LPG/Electricity/Kerosene/Wood/Others, specify _____
Open space around the house	Absent/Present
Stagnant water around the house	Absent/Present
Street road	Tar/Cement/Mud/Others
Street light	Absent/Present

Modern sanitation facility
  Drainage system
  Sewage system
	
	Yes/No
	Yes/No

Drainage System	Closed/Open
Refuse Disposal	Open dumping/Composting/Burning/Municipality collection/Community bins/Others, specify _____
Domestic animal	Absent/If present—Dog/Cow/Buffalo/Goat/Camel/Others, specify _____
Separate cattle shed (for the house with domestic animals)	Yes/No
Domestic birds/Poultry	Absent/If present—Hen/Cock/Parrot/Others, specify _____
Separate poultry shed/cage (for the house with domestic birds)	Yes/No
Rodents	Absent/If present—Rat/Others, specify _____
Street animals	Absent/If present—Dogs/Cats/Cows/Others, specify _____
Insect vectors	Absent/If present—Mosquitoes/Flies/Ticks/Others, specify _____

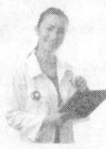

SOCIOECONOMIC STATUS

Social class/Socioeconomic status (according to rural/urban socioeconomic scale, Refer to Annexures)

VULNERABLE/TARGET GROUPS IN THE FAMILY

Total eligible couples _____   Children (0–1 years) _____   Adolescent Girls _____

Total postnatal mothers _____   Children (1–3 years) _____   Elderly (above 60 years) _____

Total antenatal mothers _____   Children (3–5 years) _____   Other, specify _____

MONTHLY FAMILY BUDGET

Income			Expenditure		
Sources	Income (In ₹)	Income (In Percentage)	Sources	Expenditure (In ₹)	Expenditure (In Percentage)
Salary			House Rent		
Rent			Education		
Agriculture			Food		
Animals			Fuel (LPG)		
Pension			Fuel (Petrol/Diesel)		
Stipend			Clothing		
Part time business			Entertainment		
Others			Electricity		
			Water		
			Property Taxes		
			Telephone/Internet		
			Transportation		
			Health		
			Festival		
			Saving		
			Insurance		
			Others		
Total (₹)			Total (₹)		

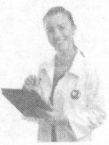

FAMILY DIETARY PATTERN

Food group	Food item	Food consumption (Yes/No)	Frequency of consumption (servings per day or per week)	Method/Form of food preparation (boiling/steaming/raw/ pressure cooking/ frying/germination etc.)	Method of food storage at home (Hygienic-H/ Unhygienic-U)
Energy giving foods	Rice				
	Wheat				
	Tubers				
	Edible oil				
	Ghee				
	Butter				
Body building foods	Meat				
	Fish				
	Poultry				
	Eggs				
	Pulses				
Protective foods	Vegetables				
	Fruits				
	Milk & milk products				
Beverages	Tea				
	Coffee				
	Water				
Others	Junk food				

SOCIOCULTURAL ASPECTS

Menstruation _____

_____

_____

_____

_____

_____

Antenatal Care _____

_____

_____

_____

_____

_____

Child Birth _____

_____

_____

_____

_____

_____

Postnatal Care _____

_____

_____

_____

_____

Care of Sick _____

_____

_____

_____

_____

_____

Food Consumption _____

_____

_____

_____

_____

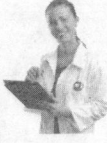

FAMILY PLANNING STATUS (ELIGIBLE COUPLE)

S. No.	Name of the eligible couple (Mr. _____ Mrs _____)	Age (yrs.)/ Sex (Male-M Female-F)	Family Planning Practice a) Yes b) No	If yes, then							
				Temporary Family Planning Method					Permanent Family Planning Method		Month and year of adoption/ Duration of use
				Condom	Oral pills	Copper-T	Inject able	Implant	Tubectomy	Vasectomy	
1.											
2.											
3.											
4.											

IMMUNIZATION STATUS

Age Group	Weeks/ Months/Years	Current Vaccine Under UIP (2017)	Child Name/Vaccines/Date of administration (D.O.A.)					
			Child -1_____		Child -2_____		Child -3_____	
			Vaccines	D.O.A.	Vaccines	D.O.A.	Vaccines	D.O.A.
Infant	At birth	BCG, OPV-0, Hep-B birth dose						
	6 weeks	OPV-1, Rota-1, Pentavalent-1, IPV-1, PCV-1						
	10 weeks	OPV-2, Rota-2, Pentavalent-2						
	14 weeks	OPV-3, Rota-3, Pentavalent-3, IPV-2, PCV-2						
	9 months	MR/Measles-1, Vit-A*, JE-1#, PCV-Booster						
Under five Children	16-24 months	DPT-Booster-1, OPV-Booster, MR/Measles-2, JE-2#						
School Going	5-6 Years	DPT-Booster -2						
Adolescent	10 years	TT-1						
	16 years	TT-2						
Pregnancy		TT-1						
		TT-2						

*Vitamin A to be given every 6 months till five years of age and a separate chart is given below for documentation. #JE vaccine given in selected districts. **BCG:** Bacillus Calmette-Guerin; **Pentavalent [DPT:** diphtheria-pertussis-tetanus; **Hep B:** Hepatitis B; **Hib:**Haemophilus influenzae type b]; **JE:** Japanese Encephalitis; **MR/Measles/MMR:** Measles Mumps rubella; **OPV:** oral polio vaccine; **TT:** tetanus toxoid; **IPV:** inactivated poliovirus vaccine. **Rota-** Rotavirus vaccine, **PCV:** Pneumonia; Additional

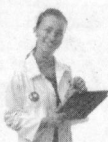

Age (in months) →		9	18	24	30	36	42	48	54	60
Dose →		1st	2nd	3rd	4th	5th	6th	7th	8th	9th
Vitamin-A Solution (D.O.A.)	Child-1 _____									
	Child-2 _____									
	Child-3 _____									

VITAL EVENTS IN THE FAMILY DURING THE LAST ONE YEAR

Birth (if any)

S. No.	Name	Date of Birth	Sex	Parents Name	Place of Birth	Birth registration- Yes/No
1.						
2.						
3.						

Death (if any)

S. No.	Name	Date of Death	Age/ Sex	Cause of Death	Place of Death	Death registration- Yes/No
1.						
2.						
3.						

Marriage (if any)

S. No.	Name of the couple	Age		Date of marriage	Marriage registration- Yes/No
		Wife	Husband		
1.					
2.					
3.					

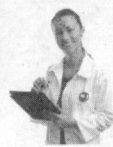

Family Health Profile

Instructions

1. Select a key case from the family—elderly, adult woman, adolescent, antenatal, postnatal, newborn, under five, physically challenged, sick, vulnerable or specific group as per assigned family priority health need.
2. Eight blank pages are provided to prepare the health profile of family members.
3. In these blank pages include family members identification data, health history, specific physical assessment, lab investigations, medications, diet chart, identified health needs/problems, and disease condition (book picture) etc.

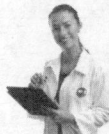

Identified Health Problems/Needs

_____
_____
_____
_____
_____
_____
_____

Prioritization of Health Problems/Needs

_____
_____
_____
_____
_____
_____
_____
_____

Priority Nursing Diagnosis

_____
_____
_____
_____
_____
_____
_____
_____
_____
_____
_____

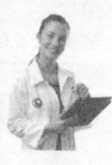

FAMILY HEALTH NURSING CARE PLAN

Assessment	Diagnosis	Goal/ Objective	Planning	Implementation	Evaluation

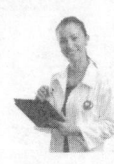

FAMILY HEALTH NURSING CARE PLAN

Assessment	Diagnosis	Goal/ Objective	Planning	Implementation	Evaluation

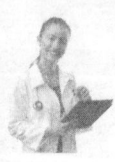

FAMILY HEALTH NURSING CARE PLAN

Assessment	Diagnosis	Goal/ Objective	Planning	Implementation	Evaluation

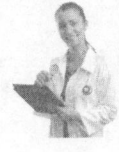

FAMILY HEALTH NURSING CARE PLAN

Assessment	Diagnosis	Goal/ Objective	Planning	Implementation	Evaluation

HEALTH EDUCATION

REFERENCES

Signature of Student

Signature of Supervisor

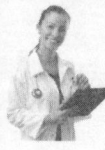

4. Health Assessment

4.1. Under Five

IDENTIFICATION DATA

Name of Child: _____

Age/Sex: _____

Name of Father: _____

Name of Mother: _____

Address: _____

Religion: Hindu/Muslims/Sikh/Christian/Others Caste-GEN/SC/ST/OBC

Occupation of father: Unemployed/government/private job/self -employed/daily wage worker/others: _____

_____

Occupation of mother: Government/private job/Self-Employed/daily wage worker/homemaker/others _____

_____

Language known: Hindi/English/Others: _____

Family size (Total Members): _____

Family Type: Nuclear/Joint: _____

Monthly Family Income: _____

Family income per capita: _____

Nearby Sub-center/PHC/CHC/District Hospital: _____

_____

Nearby Anganwadi Center: _____

Classification/Diagnosis: _____

_____

BRIEF HISTORY

History of Present Complaints

(Character/onset/location/duration/severity pattern/associated factors/medication and treatment) _____

_____

_____

_____

_____

Past Health (Medical/Surgical) History

(Antenatal history/intra-natal history/postnatal history/congenital anomaly/problems at birth/infancy//childhood/immunization/allergies (food/medication/others)/medical illness (e.g. hereditary/communicable disease/any surgery and reason/other history) _____

_____

_____

_____

_____

_____

_____

Personal and Social History

Feeding of child- colostrum/breast feed/top feed with bottle or spoon/weaning and normal diet (when started or stopped)/ food habits/feeding skills/food likes/dislikes

_____

_____

_____

_____

Type and duration of play/socialization/sleep (somnambulism/hypersomnia/night terrors/night mares)

_____

_____

_____

Habits (thumb sucking/nail biting/teeth grinding/tics/temper tantrums/head banging/pica/breath holding/nose picking/ biting)

_____

_____

_____

_____

Elimination (frequency/bladder control/bed wetting/encopresis)

_____

_____

_____

_____

Relationship with sibling and parents

_____

_____

_____

_____

School/Anganwadi/Crutch—attitude/behavior/performance of the child

_____

_____

_____

_____

_____

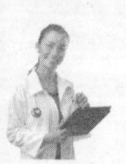

FAMILY COMPOSITION AND CHARACTERISTICS

S. No.	Name of the family members	Relationship with head of the family	Date of birth/sex (Male-M/Female-F/ Transgender-T)	Marital status (Unmarried/ married)	Educational status	Occupation	Monthly income (₹)	Dietary habits (veg/non-veg)	Addiction (smoking/ alcohol/ drugs/ others)	Health status (healthy/ unhealthy)
1.										
2.										
3.										
4.										
5.										
6.										
7.										
8.										

Family Tree/Genogramme

Key

HOUSING STANDARDS AND ENVIRONMENTAL CONDITIONS

Characteristic	Parameters
Type of house	Pucca/Semi pucca/Katcha
Total number of living room	1/2/3/4/5/6/7/8/ _____
Ventilation	Adequate (doors and windows facing each other in each room) Inadequate (doors and windows not facing each other in each room)
Bathroom	Not available/If available—Own/Public
Latrine	Not available/If available—Own/Public
Electricity	Not available/Available
Drinking water supply	Tap/Well/Lake/Pond/Others, specify _____
Kitchen	Separate/Corner of the room/Others, specify_____
Type of fuel used	LPG/Electricity/Kerosene/Wood/Others, specify _____

Modern sanitation facility
    Drainage system
    Sewage system
	
	Yes/No
	Yes/No

Drainage system	Closed/Open
Refuse disposal	Open dumping/Composting/Burning/Municipality collection/Community bins/Others, specify _____
Domestic animal	Not present/If present—Dog/Cow/Buffalo/Goat/Camel/Others, specify _____
Separate cattle shed (for the house with domestic animals)	Yes/No
Rodents	Not present/If yes—Rat/Others, specify _____
Street animals	Not present/If yes—Dogs/Cats/Cows/Others, specify _____
Insect vectors	Not present/If yes—Mosquitoes/Flies/Ticks/Others, specify _____

Recreation facilities: Market/playgrounds/cinema halls/clubs/public library/fairs
Communication facilities: Telephone connection/mobile phone/internet facility/letters
Transport facilities: Bus/auto rickshaw/taxi/four wheeler/two wheeler/train/airway
Religious places: Temple/Mosque/Gurudwara/Church

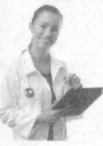

PHYSICAL EXAMINATION (put a tick (✓) mark wherever necessary or mention the finding in the provided space if needed)

General Appearance

Consciousness: Conscious/semi-conscious/unconscious
Nourishment: Well-nourished/under nourished
Activity: Active/dull/lethargic
Dress/grooming: Well-groomed/dirty
Gait (ability to walk/move): Normal/unsteady/any limp

Anthropometric Measurement

Weight: _____ kg   Length (Till 2 Years)/Height: _____ cm

MAC: _____ cm CC: _____ cm   HC: _____ cm

Degree of Malnutrition

$$\text{Weight for Age} = \frac{\text{Actual weight}}{\text{Expected weight}} \times 100 = \underline{\hspace{1cm}}$$

Classification according to IAP

Weight for Age	Classification of under nutrition	In child
≥80%	Normal	
71–80%	Grade-I	
61–70%	Grade-II	
51–60%	Grade-III	
≤50%	Grade-IV	

Classification according to WHO Growth Chart

Weight for Age (0–3 Years)

Normal	Moderately Underweight (Below -2SD to 3SD)	Severely Underweight (Below 3SD)
Yes/No	Yes/No	Yes/No

Mid Arm Circumference (7 months 60 months)

<11.5 cm (Red)	11.5–12.5 cm (Yellow)	≥12.5 cm (Green)
Yes/No	Yes/No	Yes/No

Vital Signs

Temperature: _____ °C   Pulse: _____ beats/m
Respiration: _____ breaths/m   Heart Rate: _____ beats/m

Skin Condition

Color: Normal/redness/cyanosis/jaundice/pallor/pigmented/white patches/bruise
Texture: Smooth/soft/rough/dry/wrinkled/edematous
Lesions: Absent/pustules/boil/abscess/scar/scratch marks insect bite
Turgor (elasticity): Normal/decreased

Head

Shape: Normal/Hydrocephaly/micro/macrocephaly
Scalp: Normal/injury/lump/lesion/infection
Fontanels-open/closed _____

Hair

Colour: Normal/grey/hypopigmentation
Texture: Smooth/rough/dry/oily/thin/straight/curly
Dandruff: Present/absent
Alopecia: Present/absent
Pediculosis: Present/absent
Hygiene: Good/poor

Face

Color: Normal/pale/flushed
Edema: Present/absent
Facial expression: Normal/abnormal/anxious/fear
Any malformation: _____

Eyes

Eye	Right	Left
Discharge: Present/absent		
Eyebrows: Normal/sparse/absent/meet in midline		
Eyelids: Normal/edema/ptosis/epicanthal folds		
Eyelashes: Normal/long and curly/scanty/absent/stye/infection		
Eyeball: Normal/protruded/sunken		
Sclera: Normal/jaundice/redness		
Conjunctiva: Normal/moist/pale/dryred/watery/purulent/scarring		
Pupils: Cloudy/dilated/constricted/reacting to light		
Vision: Normal/impaired/using glasses		
Movement: Normal/strabismus		

Ears

Ear	Right	Left
Position: Alignment with outer canthus of the eyes/low set		
External ear: Discharge/earwax accumulation/pain/itching		
Auditory canal: Smooth/pink/redness/discharge/wax plug/lesion/foreign body		
Tympanic membrane: Intact/redness/swelling/perforated/bulging		
Gross hearing: Normal/impaired/using hearing aid		

contd...

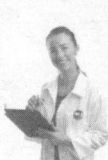

Nose

Nares: Clean/discharge/crust/blocked/foreign body/blood clots

Nasal septum: Intact/perforated/deviation _____

Mucous membrane: Normal (moist and red)/lesion/discharge/swollen/bleeding

Polyp: Present/absent

Flaring: Present/absent

Mouth

Odor: Normal/foul smelling

Malformation: Absent/cleft lip/cleft palate/unusual high arch of palate

Lips: Normal (pink, moist, smooth)/dry/cracked/cyanosis/swelling/redness/crust/cheilosis

Gums: Normal (pink and smooth)/swelling/bleeding/pus/gingivitis

Mucus membrane: Normal (pink and moist)/ulceration/white plaques/redness/lesion/koplik's spot

Tongue: Normal (pink and moist)/large/small/tongue tie/dry/coated/pallor/ulcer/redness/fissures

Teeth: normal/poor alignment/missing/dental caries/plaque/discoloration. _____

Tonsils: Normal (small, pink, symmetrical)/inflammation/enlarged/lesion/exudates/grey-yellow membrane

Throat and pharynx: Normal/redness/pus/lesion/exudate

Neck

Size: Normal/short

Lymph nodes: Non-palpable/enlarge/tender

Thyroid gland: Normal (soft and elastic)/asymmetrical/enlarge/lump/bulging

Movement (flexion/extension/rotation): Normal/stiffness/rigidity

Chest

Shape/contour: Symmetric/asymmetric/pigeon chest

Breathing pattern: Normal/unequal chest expansion/use of accessory muscles/retractions

Breath sounds: Normal/wheezing/crackles/additional _____

_____

Sputum: Color/consistency _____

_____

Heart rate: Normal/fast/slow

Heart rhythm: Regular/irregular

Heart sounds: Normal/abnormal/additional _____

_____

Any congenital malformation _____

_____

Fainting: Absent/present

Exercise intolerance: Absent/present

Nipple position: Normal/wide apart/alignment

Nipple skin: Normal/cracked/discharge

Axilla

Axillary lymph nodes—non-palpable/mobile/enlarge/tender

Abdomen

Inspection

Shape: Symmetrical/asymmetrical/distension/observable mass/hernia/ascites

Skin: Normal/lesion/rashes/previous surgery scar/vascularity

Auscultation: Bowel sounds—present/absent

Palpation: Soft/pain/tenderness/mass/no organomegaly _____

_____

_____

Abdominal Girth _____ cm

Rectum

Rectum/Anus: Normal/rashes/excoriation/bleeding/ulcer

Any congenital malformation _____

_____

Bowel pattern: Normal/constipation/diarrhea

Worms/parasites in stool: Absent/present

Urinary Bladder

Any congenital malformation _____

Bladder pattern: Normal/painful micturition/cry during micturition/weak stream/dribbling of urine

Urine: Color/odor/frequency _____

_____

Extremities

Extremities	Right	Left
Upper Extremities		
Range of motion: Symmetrical/asymmetrical		
Fingers: Normal/polydactyly/syndactyl arachnodactyl/edema		
Palm: Pale/pink		
Nails		
Color: Pink/pale/cyanosis/yellow/transverse white lines		
Shape: Normal (convex)/spoon-shaped/beau's lines/flat/clubbed/pitted		
Hygiene: Clean/dirty/long/short		
Lower Extremities		
Range of motion: Symmetrical/asymmetrical		
Rickettsial changes: No/Knock knees/Bowed legs		
Toe/foot: Normal/polydactyly/syndactyly/arachnodactyly/club foot (Talipes)/nodule/edema/pain		
Nails		
Color: Pink/pale/cyanosis		
Shape: Normal (convex)/spoon-shaped/beau's lines/flat/clubbed/pitted		
Hygiene: Clean/dirty/long/short		

contd…

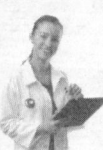

Back

Spine: Normal/kyphosis/lordosis/scoliosis/neural tube defect ___

_____

Skin: Normal/tuft of hair/masses/sacrococcygeal or anal dimple/
cyst/any discoloration _____

GENITALS

Female Genitalia

External Genitalia: Normal/congenital malformation

_____

Perineum: Normal/lesions/redness/edema/rashes

Urethra: Normal/discharge/redness/swelling

Vagina: Normal/discharge/redness/swelling

Male genitalia

External genitalia: Normal/congenital malformation

_____

Perineum: Normal/lesions/redness/edema/rashes

Foreskin: Intact/retractable/lesions

Urethral opening: Normal/epispadias/hypospadias/stenosis

Scrotum: Descended testis/undescended testis

Scrotal swelling: Absent/present

Inguinal hernia: Absent/present

Milestones (Below 2 Years)

Age	Important Skills	Remarks (achieved/not achieved/delayed, Age of achieving)
3 months	Head holding	
5–6 months	Sitting with supports	
7–8 months	Sitting without support	
10–11 months	Crawling	
9 months	Standing with support	
8–9 months	Says bisyllables words (da-da, ba-ba)	
10–12 months	Standing without support	
13–15 months	Walking without support	
12–15 months	Feeding self with spoon	
18 months	Running	
20–24 months	Climbing up stairs	

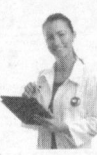

At 2 Years

Skills	Milestones	Remarks
Gross motor	Steady gait Can walk with heel-toe gait Runs more quickly Kicks large ball without falling Picks up objects from floor without losing balance	
Fine motor	Build a tower of 6-7 cubes Imitate a horizontal line or circular stroke Turns pages of book one at a time Open door by turning door knob Fold paper once	
Feeding skills	Drinks well from a small glass held in one hand Plays with food May request certain foods.	
Language	Vocabulary of 300 words 2–3 words complete sentence	
Dressing skills	Removes most of own clothes Pulls on own simple garments	
Toileting and grooming skills	Verbalize toilet needs Usually urinates when taken to the toilet May brushes teeth with help Attempts to wash self in tub	
Social Skills	Listens to stories with pictures	

At 3 Years

Skills	Milestones	Remarks
Gross motor	Walks in a straight line Walks backwards Runs without looking at first Catches ball with extended arms Kicks a ball and jumps from a height of several inches	
Fine motor	Builds tower of 9-10 cubes Copies a circle and various alphabets Can help with simple household tasks	
Dressing skills	Can put a coat without assistance Can undress self	
Feeding skills	Feeds self but with spillage Pours from a bottle	
Language	Vocabulary of 900 words 3-4 words complete sentence and ask questions	
Toileting and grooming skills	Can pull pants up and down Wash hands Can go to toilet alone Brushes teeth with help	
Social Skills	Plays simple game in parallel with other children	

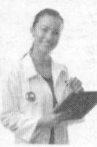

At 4 Years

Skills	Milestones	Remarks
Gross motor	Run on toe tips, balance on one foot for 3–5 seconds	
	Jumps from greater height	
	Catches ball with extended arms and with hands climbs ladder	
Fine motor	Copies a square	
	Can cut a round picture with scissors	
Feeding skills	Manage spoon with little spillage	
	Eat with fork held in finger	
Language	Vocabulary of 1500 words	
	4–5 words complete sentence, questions at peak & knows songs, poems	
Dressing skills	Can put socks with help	
	Put shoes without help	
Toileting and grooming skills	May bathe self with assistance	
	Washes and dry hands with supervision	
Social Skills	Plays in group with other children	

At 5 years

Skills	Milestones	Remarks
Gross motor	Rope and jumps over an object	
	Imitate dance steps if taught	
	Catches a ball smoothly with hands	
	Balances on one foot	
Fine motor	Copies a triangle	
	Crosses vertical lines	
	Copies letters	
	May be able to print own name	
Feeding skills	Select fork over spoon when appropriate	
Language	Vocabulary of 2100 words	
	6–8 words complete sentence, names color/days/months/pictures	
Dressing skills	May be able to tie shoe laces	
	Dress and undress self without assistance	
Toileting and grooming skills	Wipes self independently	
	Flushes toilet after each use	
	Bath self	
	Combs hairs with help	
	Can blow nose when asked	
Social skills	Domestic role play	
	Play home-home	

IMMUNIZATION STATUS

Age Group	Weeks/ Months/Years	Vaccines		Date of administration	Due date
		Under UIP	**Additional**		
Infant	At birth	BCG, OPV-0, Hep-B birth dose			
	6 weeks	OPV-1, Rota-1, Pentavalent-1, IPV-1, PCV-1			
	10 weeks	OPV-2, Rota-2, Pentavalent-2			
	14 weeks	OPV-3, Rota-3, Pentavalent-3, IPV-2, PCV-2			
	9 months	MR/Measles-1, Vit A*, JE-1#, PCV-Booster			
Under five Children	16–24 months	DPT-Booster-1, OPV-Booster, MR/Measles -2, JE-2#			

*Vitamin A to be given every 6 months till five years of age and a separate chart is provided for documentation. #JE vaccine given in selected districts.
BCG: Bacillus Calmette-Guerin; **Pentavalent [DPT:** Diphtheria-Pertussis-Tetanus; **Hep B:** Hepatitis B; **Hib:** Haemophilus influenzae type b]; **JE:** Japanese Encephalitis; **MR/Measles/MMR:** Measles Mumps Rubella; **OPV:** Oral Polio Vaccine; **TT:** Tetanus Toxoid; **IPV:** Inactivated Poliovirus Vaccine. **Rota-**Rotavirus vaccine, **PCV:** Pneumonia; Additional _____

Vitamin-A Administration

Age (in months) →	9	18	24	30	36	42	48	54	60
Dose →	1st	2nd	3rd	4th	5th	6th	7th	8th	9th
Date of administration									

Lab Investigations (if any)

S. No.	Date/time	Investigation	Patient value	Normal value	Remarks

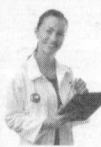

Medications (if any)

S. No.	Name and action	Dose/Route/Frequency	Indication	Side-effects

Identified Health Problems/Needs

_____
_____
_____
_____
_____

Prioritization of Health Problems/Needs

_____
_____
_____
_____
_____

Priority Nursing Diagnosis

_____
_____
_____
_____
_____

NURSING CARE PLAN

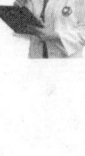

Assessment	Diagnosis	Goal/Objective	Planning	Implementation	Evaluation

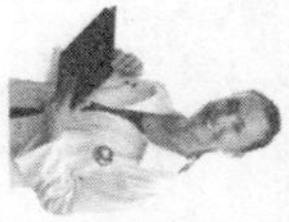

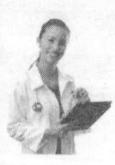

NURSING CARE PLAN

Assessment	Diagnosis	Goal/ Objective	Planning	Implementation	Evaluation

NURSING CARE PLAN

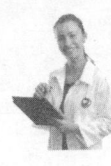

Assessment	Diagnosis	Goal/ Objective	Planning	Implementation	Evaluation

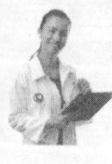

HEALTH EDUCATION

(Include diet/play/rest/immunization/hygiene/medication and its side effects/follow-up)

_____
_____
_____
_____
_____
_____
_____
_____
_____
_____
_____
_____
_____
_____
_____
_____
_____
_____
_____
_____

REFERENCES

_____
_____
_____
_____
_____
_____
_____

Signature of Student

Signature of Supervisor

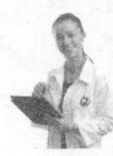

GROWTH CHART – BOY (0-3 YEARS)

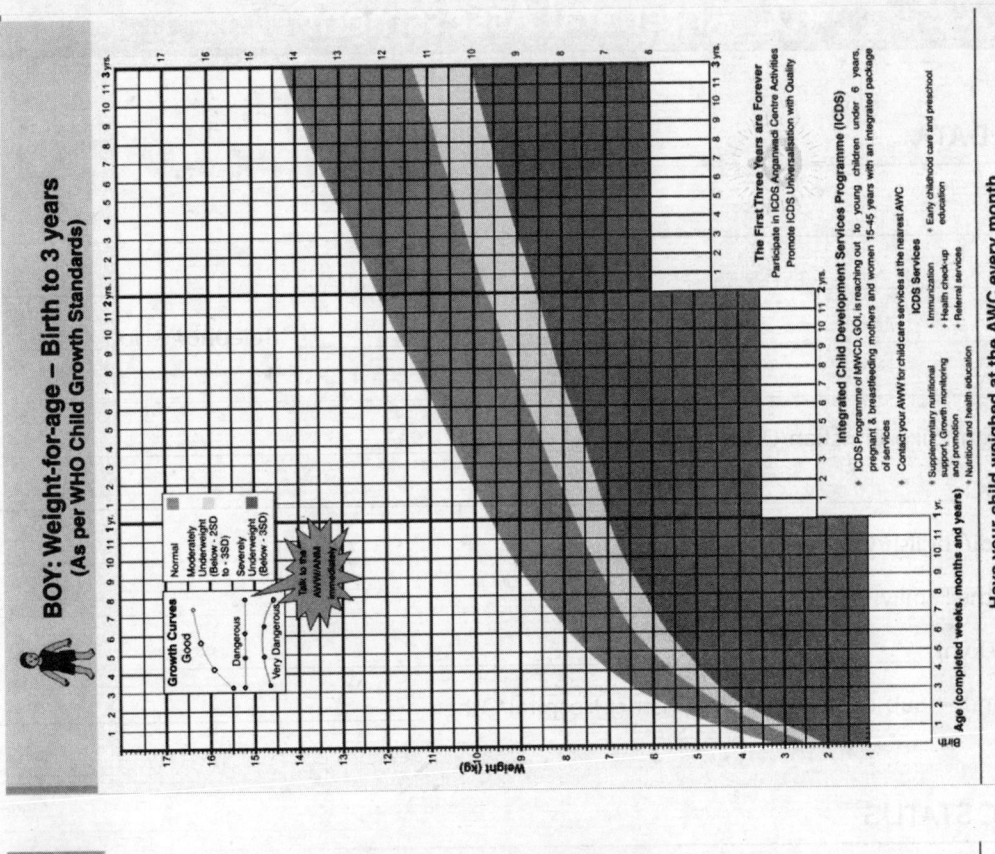

BOY: Weight-for-age – Birth to 3 years
(As per WHO Child Growth Standards)

Have your child weighed at the AWC every month

GROWTH CHART – GIRL (0-3 YEARS)

GIRL: Weight-for-age – Birth to 3 years
(As per WHO Child Growth Standards)

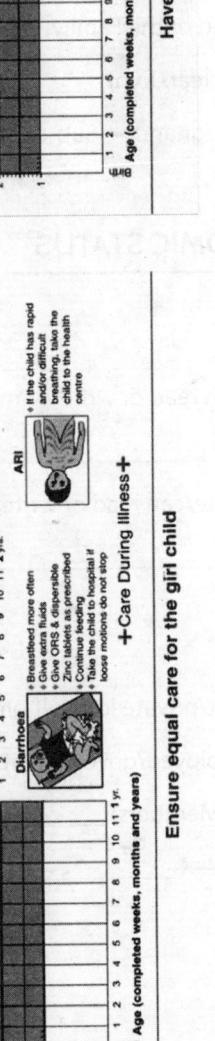

Ensure equal care for the girl child

135

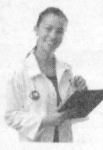

4.2. Antenatal Assessment

IDENTIFICATION DATA

Name of the Mother: _____

Husband Name: _____

Address: _____ Telephone No.: _____

Age-Self: _____ Husband: _____

Religion—Hindu/Muslims/Sikh/Christian/Others: _____

Caste—GEN/SC/ST/OBC: _____

Language known: Hindi/English/Others: _____

Relation with Head of the Family: _____

Family Type—nuclear/Joint: _____

Registration of Pregnancy—Sub-center/PHC/CHC/District Hospital/Other: _____

SOCIOECONOMIC STATUS

Education

Self—illiterate/can read or write/primary/middle/matric/senior secondary/graduate/others _____

_____

Husband—illiterate/can read or write/primary/middle/matric/senior secondary/graduate/others_____

_____

Occupation

Self—government/private job/self-employed/daily wage worker/homemaker/others _____

Husband—unemployed/government/private job/self-employed/daily wage worker/others _____

Family size (Total Members) _____ Monthly family income—₹_____

Per capita income—₹_____

FAMILY COMPOSITION AND CHARACTERISTICS

S. No.	Name of the family members	Relationship with head of the family	Date of birth/sex (Male-M/Female-F/ Transgender-T)	Marital status (Unmarried/ married)	Educational status	Occupation	Monthly income (₹)	Dietary habits (veg/non-veg)	Addiction (smoking/ alcohol/ drugs/ others)	Health status (healthy/ unhealthy)
1.										
2.										
3.										
4.										
5.										
6.										
7.										
8.										

Family Tree/Genogramme

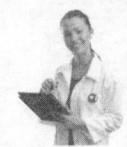

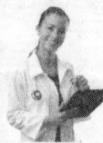

HOUSING STANDARDS AND ENVIRONMENTAL CONDITIONS

Characteristic	Parameters
Type of house	Pucca/Semi pucca/Katcha
Total number of living room	1/2/3/4/5/6/7/8/ _____
Ventilation	Adequate (doors and windows facing each other in each room) Inadequate (doors and windows not facing each other in each room)
Bathroom	Not available/If available—Own/Public
Latrine	Not available/If available—Own/Public
Electricity	Not available/Available
Drinking water supply	Tap/Well/Lake/Pond/Others, specify _____
Kitchen	Separate/Corner of the room/Others, specify_____
Type of fuel used	LPG/Electricity/Kerosene/Wood/Others, specify _____
Modern sanitation facility Drainage system Sewage system	 Yes/No Yes/No
Drainage System	Closed/Open
Refuse Disposal	Open dumping/Composting/Burning/Municipality collection/Community bins/Others, specify _____
Domestic animal	Not present/If present—Dog/Cow/Buffalo/Goat/Camel/Others, specify _____
Separate cattle shed (for the house with domestic animals)	Yes/No
Rodents	Not present/If yes—Rat/Others, specify _____
Street animals	Not present/If yes—Dogs/Cats/Cows/Others, specify _____
Insect vectors	Not present/If yes—Mosquitoes/Flies/Ticks/Others, specify _____

Recreation facilities: Market/playgrounds/cinema halls/clubs/public library/fairs

Communication facilities: Telephone connection/mobile phone/internet facility/letters

Transport facilities: Bus/auto rickshaw/taxi/four wheeler/two wheeler/train/airway

Religious places: Temple/Mosque/Gurudwara/Church

GENERAL HISTORY

Past History of Medical/Surgical illness (Yes/No)

Heart disease:	Epilepsy:	HIV/AIDS:
Renal disease:	Allergy:	RTI/STD:
Thyroid disorders:	Jaundice:	Blood transfusion:
Hypertension:	Tuberculosis:	Mental illness:
Diabetes:	Rheumatic fever:	
Asthma:	Malaria:	

Any surgery: _____

Specify if any other condition: _____

Treatment (drugs/dose/route/action): _____

FAMILY HISTORY

Family History of any illness (Yes/No)

Diabetes: Hypertension: Genetic disorders:

Multiple births: Tuberculosis:

Mental illness: Congenital abnormalities:

Any other specify:_____

ADDICTIONS (YES/NO)

Smoking: Drugs: Alcohol: Tobacco:

Any other specify:_____

PERSONAL HISTORY

Dietary habits (vegetarian/non-vegetarian/eggetarian):_____

Bowel habit (regular/irregular, stool frequency and consistency): _____

Bladder habit (regular/irregular, frequency): _____

TT immunization (dose/route/site/action): _____

IFA supplementation (dose/route/action): _____

Rest/sleep/activity/exercise/travel: _____

MENSTRUAL HISTORY

Age at menarche: _____ years   Menstruation: Regular/Irregular   Length of cycle: _____ days

Duration of blood flow: _____ days   Dysmenorrhea: Present/Absent   Leucorrhea: Present/Absent

Menorrhagia: Present/Absent

MARITAL HISTORY

Age at marriage _____ yrs   Duration of marriage _____ yrs

Consanguineous marriage—Yes/No   Relationship with husband-satisfactory/unsatisfactory

Contraceptives used: No/Condom/Cu-T/Oral contraceptive Pills/any other _____

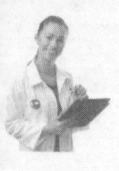

PREVIOUS OBSTETRIC HISTORY

S. No.	Date (Month/year)	Any antenatal complication & its treatment	Outcome (Abortion/ Preterm/ Full term delivery)	Mode/ Type of delivery (Normal/ Assisted/ LSCS)	Place of Delivery (Hospital/ Home)	Delivery conducted by (Doctor/ Nurse/ Dai/Other)	Condition of the child at birth (Alive/ still birth)	Sex/ Birth-weight (in kg)	Any adverse perinatal outcome & its treatment	Later Condition of the child
1.										
2.										
3.										
4.										
5.										
6.										

Gravida: _____   Parity: _____

LMP: _____   EDD: _____   POG: _____ Weeks

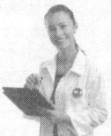

PRESENT OBSTETRIC HISTORY: MINOR DISORDERS/DISCOMFORTS (YES/NO)

Skin Pallor	Digestive system	Cardiovascular system	Micturition
Conjunctiva-	Normal-	Palpitation-	Normal-
Nails-	Heart burn (pyrosis)-	Syncope/supine hypotension-	Painful-
Tongue-	Nausea-	Varicose veins-	Scanty-
Oral mucosa-	Vomiting-	Ankle edema-	Frequent-
Palms-	Constipation-	Headache-	Incontinence-
	Diarrhea-	Fatigue-	Retention-
	Hemorrhoids-		
Jaundice	**Vision**	**Pain-**	**Discharge P/V-**
Sclera-	Normal-	Abdominal-	Red-
Skin-	Blurred-	Back-	Yellow-
Mucus membrane of mouth-		Extremities (cramps)-	White-
		Carpel tunnel Syndrome-	Thick-
		Appendicular-	Watery-
		Renal-	
Nervous system-	**Respiratory system**		
Headache-	Normal-		
Sleeplessness-	Dyspnea-		
Giddiness-	Nasal stuffiness-		

If any other, specify: _____

Sign and symptoms of associated Medical/surgical illness: _____

_____

Treatment (drugs/dose/route/action): _____

_____

LAB INVESTIGATIONS

S. No.	Date	Investigation	Patient value	Normal Value	Remarks
		Blood test			
		Hb/dl-			
		Blood group/Rh- Self Husband			
		Hbs Ag			
		Blood sugar- Fasting			
		Post Prandial			
		HIV			
		VDRL- Self			
		Husband			
		Urine test- Albumin (protein)			
		Sugar			
		USG			

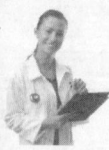

GENERAL PHYSICAL EXAMINATIONS

Height (cm): _____   Weight (kg): _____   Built- obese/average/thin   Weight gain (kg): _____

Vitals

Temperature: _____ °C   Pulse: _____ beats/m   Respiration _____ breaths/m   BP _____ mm Hg

HEAD TO FOOT ASSESSMENT

General appearance—lethargic/sick/active/anemic/pallor _____

Stature—normal/short _____

Skin condition—hydrated/dehydrated _____

Skin pigmentation—absent/If present-face/breast/abdomen/other _____

Striae—absent/If present-breast/abdomen/thigh/upper arm/other _____

Hair—normal/rough/dry/oily/thin/dandruff/pediculosis/poor hygiene _____

Facial expression—normal/lethargic/pale/confused _____

Eyes—normal/puffiness/blurred vision/blindness/jaundice/pallor _____

Nose—normal/nasal polyps/epistaxis/nasal stuffiness/nasal septum deviation/rhinitis _____

Lips—normal (pink, moist, smooth)/dry/cracked/cyanosis/swelling/redness/crust/cheilosis Tongue—normal (pink and moist)/pale/dry/coated/redness/lesion/swelling/glossitis _____

Gums—normal (pink and smooth)/swelling/bleeding/pus/gingivitis _____

Teeth—normal/poor alignment/missing/dental caries/plaque/discoloration _____

Ear—normal/discharge/earwax accumulation/lesion/foreign body/pain/itching/tinnitus/hearing aid _____

Neck—symmetrical/lymphedenopathy/thyroid enlargement _____

Breast—normal/prominent Montgomery's tubercles/presence of secondary areola/tingling sensation/tenderness/fullness

Nipples—normal/inverted/flat/crack/dry _____

Nipple size—normal/big/small _____

Colostrum—absent/thick yellow/thin/watery _____

Hands—normal/edema/bony deformity/capillary refill time _____ sec

Perineal hygiene—good/poor _____

Vagina—normal/discharge/bleeding/infection/boils _____

Rectum and anus—normal/diarrhea/constipation/hemorrhoids _____

Legs—normal/varicose veins/edema/bony deformity _____

Back—symmetrical spine/presence of rhomboid of machales/deformity _____

Lymph node enlargement—absent/If present—neck/axilla/groin/abdomen/other _____

Edema—absent/If present—face/peri-orbital/hands/legs/feet/ankle/vulva/abdomen/other _____

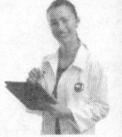

ABDOMINAL EXAMINATION

Inspection	Palpation	Auscultation
Shape of abdomen—round/spherical	Fundal height_____ cm _____wks	FHS—_____/min
Linea nigra—dark/light	Abdominal girth (cm)—	Rhythm—regular/irregular
Striae gravidum—pink/silver/purple	Presentation—	
Previous surgery scar—present/absent	Fetal positions—	
	Lie—longitudinal/transeverse/oblique	
	Engagement—Engaged/not engaged	

PROBLEMS/DANGER SIGNS REQUIRING URGENT REFERRAL

Problems	Yes/No	Remarks
Temperature more than 38°C		
Persistence/excessive vomiting		
Breathlessness at rest		
Fast or difficulty breathing		
Malpresentation		
Multiple pregnancy		
Any abnormal discharge/bleeding P/V during pregnancy		
High BP (>140/90 mm Hg) with proteins in the urine, and severe headache with blurred vision or epigastric pain		
Hemoglobin <7 g%		
Convulsions or loss of consciousness		
Decreased or absent foetal movements		
Continuous severe abdominal pain		
FHR >160/minute or <120/minute		

Any Abnormal Signs Detected

_____

_____

_____

_____

_____

_____

_____

_____

Health Problems/Needs Identified

_____
_____
_____
_____
_____
_____
_____
_____

Prioritization of Health Problems/Needs

_____
_____
_____
_____
_____
_____
_____
_____
_____
_____

Priority Nursing Diagnosis

_____
_____
_____
_____
_____
_____
_____
_____
_____

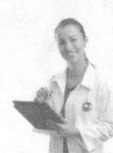

NURSING CARE PLAN

Assessment	Diagnosis	Goal/ Objective	Planning	Implementation	Evaluation

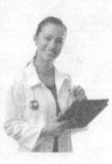

NURSING CARE PLAN

Assessment	Diagnosis	Goal/ Objective	Planning	Implementation	Evaluation

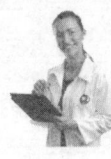

NURSING CARE PLAN

Assessment	Diagnosis	Goal/Objective	Planning	Implementation	Evaluation

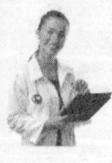

HEALTH EDUCATION

(Antenatal visit/diet/IFA supplementation/TT immunization/normal physiological changes/minor disorders/sex/travel/exercise/rest/self-care/hygiene/Daily Fetal Movement Records/warning signs/preparation for confinement)

_____
_____
_____
_____
_____
_____
_____
_____
_____
_____
_____
_____
_____
_____
_____
_____
_____

REFERENCES

_____
_____
_____
_____
_____
_____

Signature of Student   **Signature of Supervisor**

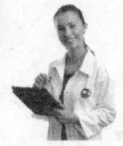

4.3. Postnatal Assessment

IDENTIFICATION DATA

Name of the Mother: _____

Husband Name: _____

Address: _____ Telephone No.:_____

Age—Self: _____ Husband: _____

Religion—Hindu/Muslims/Sikh/Christian/Others: _____

Caste—GEN/SC/ST/OBC: _____

Language known—Hindi/English/Others: _____

Relation with Head of the Family: _____

Family Type—Nuclear/Joint: _____

Date of delivery: _____

Delivered at—Sub-center/PHC/CHC/District Hospital/Other: _____

SOCIOECONOMIC STATUS

Education

Self—illiterate/can read or write/primary/middle/matric/senior secondary/graduate/others _____

_____

Husband—illiterate/can read or write/primary/middle/matric/senior secondary/graduate/others_____

_____

Occupation

Self—government/private job/self-employed/daily wage worker/homemaker/others _____

Husband—unemployed/government/private job/self-employed/daily wage worker/others _____

Family size (Total Members) _____ Monthly family income—₹_____

Per capita income—₹ _____

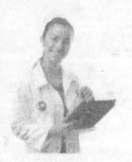

FAMILY COMPOSITION AND CHARACTERISTICS

S. No.	Name of the family members	Relationship with head of the family	Date of birth/sex (Male-M/Female-F/Transgender-T)	Marital status (Unmarried/married)	Educational status	Occupation	Monthly income (₹)	Dietary habits (veg/non-veg)	Addiction (smoking/ alcohol/ drugs/ others)	Health status (healthy/ unhealthy)
1.										
2.										
3.										
4.										
5.										
6.										
7.										
8.										

Key

Family Tree/Genogramme

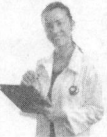

HOUSING STANDARDS AND ENVIRONMENTAL CONDITIONS

Characteristic	Parameters
Type of house	Pucca/Semi pucca/Katcha
Total number of living room	1/2/3/4/5/6/7/8/ _____
Ventilation	Adequate (doors and windows facing each other in each room) Inadequate (doors and windows not facing each other in each room)
Bathroom	Not available/If available—Own/Public
Latrine	Not available/If available—Own/Public
Electricity	Not available/Available
Drinking water supply	Tap/Well/Lake/Pond/Others, specify _____
Kitchen	Separate/Corner of the room/Others, specify _____
Type of fuel used	LPG/Electricity/Kerosene/Wood/Others, specify _____
Modern sanitation facility Drainage system Sewage system	 Yes/No Yes/No
Drainage system	Closed/Open
Refuse disposal	Open dumping/Composting/Burning/Municipality collection/Community bins/Others, specify _____
Domestic animal	Not present/If present—Dog/Cow/Buffalo/Goat/Camel/Others, specify _____
Separate cattle shed (for the house with domestic animals)	Yes/No
Rodents	Not present/If yes—Rat/Others, specify _____
Street animals	Not present/If yes—Dogs/Cats/Cows/Others, specify _____
Insect vectors	Not present/If yes—Mosquitoes/Flies/Ticks/Others, specify _____

Recreation facilities: Market/playgrounds/cinema halls/clubs/public library/fairs
Communication facilities: Telephone connection/mobile phone/internet facility/letters
Transport facilities: Bus/auto rickshaw/taxi/four wheeler/two wheeler/train/airway
Religious places: Temple/Mosque/Gurudwara/Church

GENERAL HISTORY

Past History of Medical/Surgical illness (Yes/No)

Heart disease:	Epilepsy:	HIV/AIDS:
Renal disease:	Allergy:	RTI/STD:
Thyroid disorders:	Jaundice:	Blood transfusion:
Hypertension:	Tuberculosis:	Mental illness:
Diabetes:	Rheumatic fever:	
Asthma:	Malaria:	

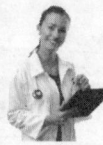

Any surgery: _____

Specify if any other condition: _____

Drugs and treatment: _____

FAMILY HISTORY

Family History of any illness (Yes/No)

Diabetes:	Hypertension:	Any other specify
Multiple births:	Tuberculosis:	_____
Mental illness:	Congenital abnormalities:	_____
Hypertension:		

ADDICTIONS (YES/NO)

Smoking: Drugs: Alcohol: Tobacco:

Any other specify:_____

PERSONAL HISTORY

Dietary habits (vegetarian/non-vegetarian/eggetarian):_____

Bowel habit (regular/irregular, stool frequency and consistency): _____

Bladder habit (regular/irregular, frequency): _____

TT immunization (dose/route/site/action): _____

IFA supplementation (dose/route/action): _____

Rest/sleep/activity/exercise/travel: _____

MENSTRUAL HISTORY

Age at menarche: _____ years	Menstruation: Regular/Irregular	Length of cycle: _____ days
Duration of blood flow: _____ days	Dysmenorrhea: Present/Absent	Leucorrhea: Present/Absent
Menorrhagia: Present/Absent		

MARITAL HISTORY

Age at marriage _____ yrs   Duration of marriage _____ yrs

Consanguineous marriage—Yes/No   Relationship with husband—satisfactory/unsatisfactory

Contraceptives used—No/Condom/Cu-T/Oral contraceptive Pills/any other _____

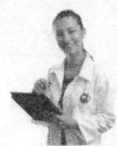

PREVIOUS OBSTETRIC HISTORY

S. No.	Date (Month/year)	Any antenatal complication & its treatment	Outcome (Abortion/Preterm/Full term delivery)	Mode/Type of delivery (Normal/Assisted/LSCS)	Place of Delivery (Hospital/Home)	Delivery conducted by (Doctor/Nurse/Dai/Other)	Condition of the child at birth (Alive/still birth)	Sex/Birth-weight (in kg)	Any adverse perinatal outcome & its treatment	Later Condition of the child
1.										
2.										
3.										
4.										
5.										
6.										

Gravida: Parity: EDD: POG: Weeks

LMP:

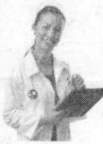

PRESENT OBSTETRIC HISTORY: MINOR DISORDERS/DISCOMFORTS (YES/NO)

Skin Pallor	Digestive system	Cardiovascular system	Micturition
Conjunctiva-	Normal-	Palpitation-	Normal-
Nails-	Heart burn (pyrosis)-	Syncope/supine hypotension-	Painful-
Tongue-	Nausea-	Varicose veins-	Scanty-
Oral mucosa-	Vomiting-	Ankle edema-	Frequent-
Palms-	Constipation-	Headache-	Incontinence-
	Diarrhea-	Fatigue-	Retention-
	Hemorrhoids-		
Jaundice	**Vision**	**Pain-**	**Discharge P/V-**
Sclera-	Normal-	Abdominal-	Red-
Skin-	Blurred-	Back-	Yellow-
Mucus membrane of mouth-		Extremities (cramps)-	White-
		Carpel tunnel syndrome-	Thick-
		Appendicular-	Watery-
		Renal-	
Nervous system-	**Respiratory system**		
Headache-	Normal-		
Sleeplessness-	Dyspnea-		
Giddiness-	Nasal stuffiness-		

If any other, specify: _____

Sign and symptoms of associated Medical/surgical illness: _____

_____

Treatment (drugs/dose/route/action): _____

_____

LAB INVESTIGATIONS

S. No.	Date	Investigation	Patient value	Normal Value	Remarks
		Blood test			
		Hb/dl-			
		Blood group/Rh- Self Husband			
		Hbs Ag			
		Blood sugar-Fasting			
		Post Prandial			
		HIV			
		VDRL- Self			
		Husband			
		Urine test-Albumin (protein)			
		Sugar			
		USG			

PRESENT DELIVERY/OPERATION HISTORY

- **Type/mode of delivery** _____

- **If normal vaginal delivery** _____

  Episiotomy-yes/no _____

  Tear-yes/no _____

- **Treatment** (drugs/dose/route/action) _____

GENERAL PHYSICAL EXAMINATIONS

Height (cm):   Weight (kg):   Built: Obese/average/thin   Weight gain (kg):

Vitals

Temperature: _____ °C   Pulse: _____beats/m   Respiration _____ breaths/m   BP _____ mm Hg

HEAD TO FOOT ASSESSMENT

General appearance—lethargic/sick/active/anemic/pallor _____

Stature—normal/short _____

Skin condition—hydrated/dehydrated _____

Skin pigmentation—absent/If present-face/breast/abdomen/other _____

Striae—absent/If present-breast/abdomen/thigh/upper arm/other _____

Hair—normal/rough/dry/oily/thin/dandruff/pediculosis/poor hygiene _____

Facial expression—normal/lethargic/pale/confused _____

Eyes—normal/puffiness/blurred vision/blindness/jaundice/pallor _____

Nose—normal/nasal polyps/epistaxis/nasal stuffiness/nasal septum deviation/rhinitis ____

Lips—normal (pink, moist, smooth)/dry/cracked/cyanosis/swelling/redness/crust/cheilosis Tongue—normal (pink and moist)/pale/dry/coated/redness/lesion/swelling/glossitis _____

Gums—normal (pink and smooth)/swelling/bleeding/pus/gingivitis _____

Teeth—normal/poor alignment/missing/dental caries/plaque/discoloration _____

Ear—normal/discharge/earwax accumulation/lesion/foreign body/pain/itching/tinnitus/hearing aid ____

Neck—symmetrical/lymphedenopathy/thyroid enlargement _____

Breast—normal/prominent Montgomery's tubercles/presence of secondary areola/tingling sensation/tenderness/fullness

Nipples—normal/inverted/flat/crack/dry _____

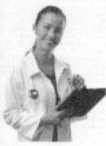

Nipple size—normal/big/small _____

Colostrum—absent/thick yellow/thin/watery _____

Hands—normal/edema/bony deformity/capillary refill time _____ sec

Perineal hygiene—good/poor _____

Vagina—normal/discharge/bleeding/infection/boils _____

Rectum and anus—normal/diarrhea/constipation/hemorrhoids _____

Legs—normal/varicose veins/edema/bony deformity _____

Back—symmetrical spine/presence of rhomboid of machales/deformity _____

Lymph node enlargement—absent/If present—neck/axilla/groin/abdomen/other _____

Edema—absent/If present—face/peri-orbital/hands/legs/feet/ankle/vulva/abdomen/other _____

ABDOMINAL EXAMINATION

Inspection	Palpation	Auscultation

Presence of scare/wound-absent/present
If LSCS scar-
   Discharge—absent/present
   Redness—absent/present
   Tenderness—absent/present
	Fundal height_____ cm _____wks
	Abdominal girth (cm)
	Consistency of uterus-hard/firm/boggy
		Bowel sound-_____/min

Mother's immunization (e.g. Anti-D): Yes/No
Personal hygiene: Bathed/brushed teeth/washed hair/clean clothes/clean perineal pad
Diet: Liquid/Semisolid/Solid/Extra ghee/Special diet
Room environment: Ventilated/Clean

PROBLEMS/DANGER SIGNS REQUIRING URGENT REFERRAL

Problems	Yes/No	Remarks
Excessive bleeding, i.e. soaking more than 2–3 pads in 20–30 minutes after delivery.		
Convulsions		
Fever		
Severs abdominal pain		
Difficulty in breathing		
Foul-smelling lochia		

Identified Health Problems/Needs

_____
_____
_____
_____
_____
_____
_____
_____

Prioritization of Health Problems/Needs

_____
_____
_____
_____
_____
_____
_____
_____

Priority Nursing Diagnosis

_____
_____
_____
_____
_____
_____
_____
_____

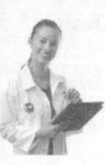

NURSING CARE PLAN

Assessment	Diagnosis	Goal/ Objective	Planning	Implementation	Evaluation

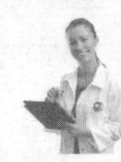

NURSING CARE PLAN

Assessment	Diagnosis	Goal/ Objective	Planning	Implementation	Evaluation

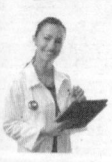

NURSING CARE PLAN

Assessment	Diagnosis	Goal/Objective	Planning	Implementation	Evaluation

HEALTH EDUCATION

(Include diet/fluids/breast and perineal care/hygiene/exercise/rest/self-care/family planning/sex/travel/medication and its side effects/follow-up)

_____

_____

_____

_____

_____

_____

_____

_____

_____

_____

_____

_____

_____

_____

_____

_____

REFERENCES

_____

_____

_____

_____

_____

_____

_____

Signature of Student

Signature of Supervisor

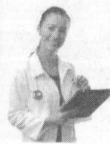

4.4. Newborn Assessment

IDENTIFICATION DATA

Name of the baby (if given): _____

Age/Sex: _____

Date/Time of Birth: _____

Name of the Mother: _____

Name of the Father: _____

Birth-weight: _____ kg

Birth order: 1/2/3/4/5/ _____

Address: _____

Type of delivery: Normal Vaginal Delivery/Assisted/LSCS/ other: _____

Place of birth: Sub-center/PHC/CHC/District Hospital/Other: _____

Gestational Age:_____ weeks [Full term (37–42 weeks)/Pre term (after 28 weeks)/Post term (after 42 weeks)]

BIRTH HISTORY

APGAR Score

S. No.	Criteria	0 Score	1 Score	2 Score
1.	Color	Pale/Blue	Body pink/Limbs blue	Completely pink
2.	Respiration	Absent	Weak cry	Good cry
3.	Heart rate	Absent	Slow (<100/min.)	>100 min.
4.	Muscle tone	Limp	Some flexion	Active movements
5.	Reflexes	Absent	Facial grimace	Crying

Total Score: At birth _____ After 5 minutes _____

0–3 Severely Depressed	4–6 Moderately Depressed	7–10 Excellent condition

IMMMUNIZATION AT BIRTH

Age Group	Time	Vaccine	Dose	Route	Site	Date and time of administration
Newborn	At birth	BCG				
		OPV-0				
		Hep-B birth dose				

BCG: Bacillus Calmette-Guerin, **Hep B:** Hepatitis B, **OPV:** oral polio vaccine

VITAL SIGNS

Temperature _____ °C   Heart rate _____ beats/min   Respiration _____ breaths/min

General Appearance

Activity—alert/lethargic or irritable/unconscious

Cry/activity—loud/poor

Bath given—yes/no

Clothing—clean/seasonal/dirty

Congenital anomaly/birth injury—absent/If present, specify _____

Feeding

Colostrums—Given/Not

Feeding started with—Breast milk/Ghutti/Honey/milk with spoon/bottle

Feeding—Well/difficulty

Feeds per day: _____

PHYSICAL EXAMINATION (put a tick (✓) mark wherever necessary or mention the finding in the provided space if needed)

Anthropometric Measurements		Ears
Head circumference:	cm	Shape/size: Normal/small/large/absent/deformed
Chest circumference:	cm	Position: Alignment with outer canthus of eye/low set
Abdominal circumference:	cm	Cartilage: Well-formed/not well-formed
Length (crown to heel):	cm	Discharge: Present/absent
Weight:	kg	Any other abnormality_____
		_____

Skin: Vernix caseosa/milia/lanugo/Mongolian spot/erythema toxicum

Color of skin: Pink/pale/jaundice/redness/if cyanosis- central (lips and tongue)/acrocynosis(palm and soles)

Infection: Absent/pustules/a big boil/abscess

Turgor: Normal/decreased

Nose

Nostrils: Patent/blocked

Discharge or lesion: Present/absent

Any other abnormality_____
_____

Head

Shape: Normocephalic/microcephalic/macrocephali/hydrocephalic

Anterior fontanels: Diamond shaped/flat/soft/firm/bulging/depressed/small/large

Posterior fontanels: Triangular shaped/flat/soft/firm/bulging/depressed/small/large

Birth changes: Absent/moulding/caput succedaneum/cephalohematoma

Hair distribution: Normal/dense/sparse

Any other abnormality_____
_____

Mouth

Cleft lip or cleft palate: Present/absent

Lips: Pink/dry/cyanosis/sucking blisters

Color of tongue: Pink/blue

Tongue tie: Present/absent

Oral thrush: Present/absent

Throat: Clear/secretions

Any other abnormality_____
_____

Eyes

Sclera color: White/yellow/red

Discharge: Absent/If present-purulent/watery _____

Tears: Present/absent

Eye lids: Normal/swollen

Any other abnormality_____

Neck

Shape: Symmetrical/asymmetrical/short

Lymph nodes: Enlarge/not enlarged

Movements: Possible/impossible

contd...

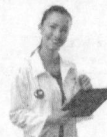

Chest:

Shape: Symmetrical/asymmetrical

Expansion: Bilateral/unilateral

Chest indrawing: Absent/mild/severe

Mark of any injury: Absent/If present, specify _____
_____

Respiratory movements: Normal/abnormal _____

Heart sound: Normal/abnormal _____

Respiratory sound: Normal/abnormal _____

Breast and nipples:

Breast: Enlarged/not enlarged

Discharge: Absent/If present, specify _____

Position: Normal/wide apart

Abdomen:

Any distension: Present/absent

Umbilical stump: Dry/healthy/redness/bleeding/pus

Bowel sounds: Present/absent

Back

Spine curvature: Normal/C-shape/arching, if any abnormality, specify _____

Skin: tuft of hair/masses/sacrococcygeal or anal dimple/cyst/any discoloration _____

Rectum and anus-patent/imperforated

Genitalia- In Male

Size of penis- short/normal (≥ 2cm)

Testes in scrotal sac– descended/undescended

Urinary meatus –central/epispadiasis/hypospadiasis/phimosis/stenosis

In Female

Labia minora and clitoris: Covered/not covered by

Labia majora.

Vaginal discharge: Absent/blood stained

Hip joints

Range of motion: Normal/abnormal

Fracture or dislocations: Present/absent

Limbs

Movement: Symmetrical/asymmetrical

Leg length discrepancy: Absent/present

Congenital deformity of digits: Absent/extra fingers/extra toes/fused digits/club foot

Palmer creases: Present/simian

Any other abnormality_____
_____

NEUROMUSCULAR SYSTEM (REFLEXES)

S. No.	Reflexes	Normal Response	Remarks (Present/Absent)
1.	Blinking or corneal reflex	Protection of the eye by rapid eye lid closure when the eyes are exposed to bright light.	
2.	Glabellar Reflex	Tap gently over the forehead the eyes will blink	
3.	Doll's Eye Reflex	When the head is turned slowly to the right or left side normally the eyes do not move	
4.	Sneezing and Coughing Reflex	When the foreign body enters into the upper and lower airways, there is clearing of upper air passage by sneezing and lower air passage by coughing.	
5.	Rooting Reflex	When the cheek or corner of the mouth is stroked, the infant head should turn towards the stimulus and the mouth should be open.	
6.	Sucking Reflex	On touching or stroking the lips, the mouth opens and sucking movement begins.	
7.	Swallowing Reflex	It accompanies the sucking as the food reaching the posterior aspect of the mouth is swallowed	

contd...

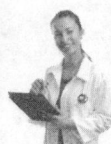

S. No.	Reflexes	Normal Response	Remarks (Present/Absent)
8.	Gagging reflex	When the posterior pharynx is stimulated with food there is an immediate return of undigested food.	
9.	Extrusion Reflex	When substance placed on anterior position of tongue will be expelled out.	
10.	Palmer Reflex	When object are placed in newborn's palm, the newborn grasps	
11.	Plantar Reflex	When the object touches the sole of foot at the base of toes, toes grasp around very small object.	
12.	Dancing and Stepping Reflex	Hold neonate in a vertical position with the feet touching a flat, firm surface, there will be rapid alternating flexion and extension as in stepping.	
13.	Babinski Reflex	Stroking the lateral aspect of the sole of foot with a relatively sharp object from heel up towards the little toe and cross the foot to the big toe, there will be fanning of toes.	
14.	Tonic Neck Reflex (fencing position)	Turning the head quickly to one side while the infant is supine, the arm and leg on the same side extends and on the opposite side flexes. Both hands may make fists.	
15.	Moro Reflex (Startle Reflex)	By the sudden movement or loud noise, there is extension and abduction of extremities with fanning of the fingers forming 'C' shape followed by flexion of extremities in embracing motion.	
16.	Crawl Reflex	When placed on abdomen newborn makes crawling movements with arms and legs.	

LAB INVESTIGATIONS (IF ANY)

S. No.	Date/time	Investigation	Infant's value	Normal Value	Remarks

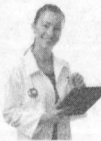

PROBLEMS REQUIRING URGENT REFERRAL

Problems	Yes/No	Remarks
Baby is not accepting the breastfeed.		
Baby looks sick (lethargic or irritable).		
Baby has fever or feels cold to the touch.		
Breathing is fast or difficult (chest indrawing).		
Baby looks yellow (palm and soles), pale or bluish.		
Baby's body is arched forward.		
Irregular movements of the body, limbs or face.		
Umbilicus is red, swolleh or draining pus.		
Baby has not passed meconium within 24 hours of birth.		
Baby has diarrhea.		
Baby has blood in the stools.		
Baby has convulsions		

Identified Health Problems/Needs

_____

_____

_____

_____

_____

Prioritization of Health Problems/Needs

_____

_____

_____

_____

_____

Priority Nursing Diagnosis

_____

_____

_____

_____

_____

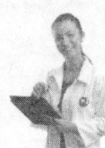

NURSING CARE PLAN

Assessment	Diagnosis	Goal/ Objective	Planning	Implementation	Evaluation

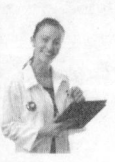

NURSING CARE PLAN

Assessment	Diagnosis	Goal/ Objective	Planning	Implementation	Evaluation

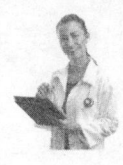

NURSING CARE PLAN

Assessment	Diagnosis	Goal/ Objective	Planning	Implementation	Evaluation

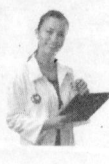

HEALTH EDUCATION

(Include breastfeeding/eye and cord care/baby bath/hygiene/seasonal clothings/prevention of hypothermia/ immunization/registration of birth/aadhar card/danger signs/follow-up)

_____

_____

_____

_____

_____

_____

_____

_____

_____

_____

_____

_____

_____

_____

_____

_____

_____

REFERENCES

_____

_____

_____

_____

_____

_____

Signature of Student   **Signature of Supervisor**

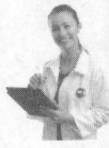

5. Health Education

5.1. Lesson Plan-1 (Individual)

ON

_____

IDENTIFICATION DATA

Name of the Health Educator: _____

Health Education Topic _____

Age Group/Participants: _____

Size of the Group: _____

Date of Teaching: _____

Time of Teaching: _____

Duration of Teaching: _____

Place of Teaching: _____

Method of Teaching: _____

Teaching Aids: _____

Medium of Teaching/Language: _____

Name of the Student's Supervisor: _____

Self-Introduction

_____

_____

_____

_____

Topic Introduction

_____

_____

_____

_____

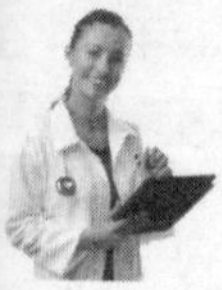

Previous Knowledge of the Group

_____

_____

_____

_____

_____

_____

_____

_____

General Objective

_____

_____

_____

_____

Specific Objectives

_____

_____

_____

_____

_____

_____

_____

_____

_____

_____

_____

_____

_____

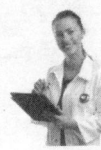

Time	Specific Objectives	Content	Health Educator Teaching Activity	A-V Aids	Participant's Evaluation

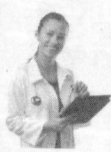

Time	Specific Objectives	Content	Health Educator Teaching Activity	A-V Aids	Participant's Evaluation

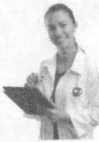

Time	Specific Objectives	Content	Health Educator Teaching Activity	A-V Aids	Participant's Evaluation

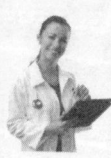

Time	Specific Objectives	Content	Health Educator Teaching Activity	A-V Aids	Participant's Evaluation

Time	Specific Objectives	Content	Health Educator Teaching Activity	A-V Aids	Participant's Evaluation

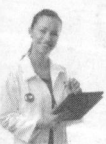

Time	Specific Objectives	Content	Health Educator Teaching Activity	A-V Aids	Participant's Evaluation

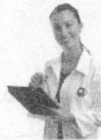

Time	Specific Objectives	Content	Health Educator Teaching Activity	A-V Aids	Participant's Evaluation

REFERENCES

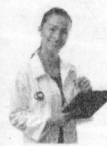

5.2. Lesson Plan-2 (Family)

ON

_____

IDENTIFICATION DATA

Name of the Health Educator: _____

Health Education Topic _____

Age Group/Participants: _____

Size of the Group: _____

Date of Teaching: _____

Time of Teaching: _____

Duration of Teaching: _____

Place of Teaching: _____

Method of Teaching: _____

Teaching Aids: _____

Medium of Teaching/Language: _____

Name of the Student's Supervisor: _____

Self-Introduction

_____

_____

_____

_____

_____

Topic Introduction

_____

_____

_____

_____

_____

Previous Knowledge of the Group

_____

_____

_____

_____

_____

_____

_____

_____

_____

General Objective

_____

_____

_____

_____

Specific Objectives

_____

_____

_____

_____

_____

_____

_____

_____

_____

_____

_____

_____

_____

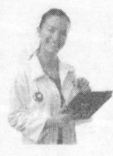

Time	Specific Objectives	Content	Health Educator Teaching Activity	A-V Aids	Participant's Evaluation

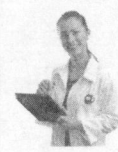

Time	Specific Objectives	Content	Health Educator Teaching Activity	A-V Aids	Participant's Evaluation

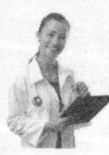

Time	Specific Objectives	Content	Health Educator Teaching Activity	A-V Aids	Participant's Evaluation

Time	Specific Objectives	Content	Health Educator Teaching Activity	A-V Aids	Participant's Evaluation

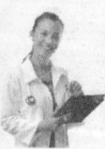

Time	Specific Objectives	Content	Health Educator Teaching Activity	A-V Aids	Participant's Evaluation

Time	Specific Objectives	Content	Health Educator Teaching Activity	A-V Aids	Participant's Evaluation

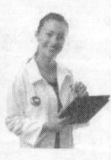

Time	Specific Objectives	Content	Health Educator Teaching Activity	A-V Aids	Participant's Evaluation

REFERENCES

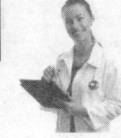

5.3. Lesson Plan-3 (Community)

ON

_____

IDENTIFICATION DATA

Name of the Health Educator: _____

Health Education Topic _____

Age Group/Participants: _____

Size of the Group: _____

Date of Teaching: _____

Time of Teaching: _____

Duration of Teaching: _____

Place of Teaching: _____

Method of Teaching: _____

Teaching Aids: _____

Medium of Teaching/Language: _____

Name of the Student's Supervisor: _____

Self-Introduction

_____

_____

_____

_____

Topic Introduction

_____

_____

_____

_____

_____

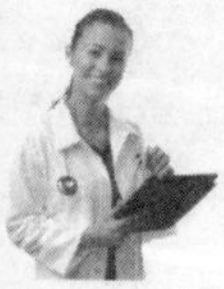

Previous Knowledge of the Group

_____
_____
_____
_____
_____
_____
_____
_____

General Objective

_____
_____
_____
_____

Specific Objectives

_____
_____
_____
_____
_____
_____
_____
_____
_____
_____
_____
_____

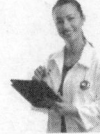

Time	Specific Objectives	Content	Health Educator Teaching Activity	A-V Aids	Participant's Evaluation

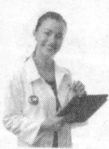

Time	Specific Objectives	Content	Health Educator Teaching Activity	A-V Aids	Participant's Evaluation

Time	Specific Objectives	Content	Health Educator Teaching Activity	A-V Aids	Participant's Evaluation

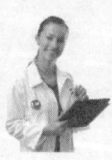

Time	Specific Objectives	Content	Health Educator Teaching Activity	A-V Aids	Participant's Evaluation

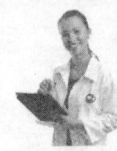

Time	Specific Objectives	Content	Health Educator Teaching Activity	A-V Aids	Participant's Evaluation

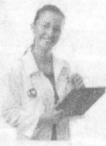

Time	Specific Objectives	Content	Health Educator Teaching Activity	A-V Aids	Participant's Evaluation

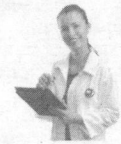

Time	Specific Objectives	Content	Health Educator Teaching Activity	A-V Aids	Participant's Evaluation

REFERENCES

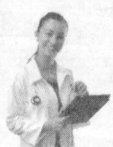

6. Nutritional Assessment

IDENTIFICATION DATA

Name: _____

Address: _____

Age/Sex: _____

Religion—Hindu/Muslims/Sikh/Christian/Others: _____

Caste—GEN/SC/ST/OBC: _____

Occupation—Unemployed/government/private job/Self-Employed/daily wage worker/homemaker/others: _____

Region—North/South/East/West: _____

Level of activity—Sedentary/moderate/heavy worker: _____

Relation with head of the family: _____

Family size (Total Members): _____

Family income per capita (₹): _____

Nearby Sub-center/PHC/CHC/District Hospital: _____

FAMILY COMPOSITION AND CHARACTERISTICS

S. No.	Name of the family members	Relationship with head of the family	Date of Birth/ Sex (Male-M/ Female-F/ Transgender-T)	Marital Status (Unmarried/ Married)	Educa- tional status	Occup- ation	Monthly income (₹)	Dietary habits (Veg/ Non-veg)	Addiction (Smoking Alcohol/ Drugs/ Others)	Health status (Healthy/ unhealthy)
1.										
2.										
3.										
4.										
5.										
6.										
7.										
8.										

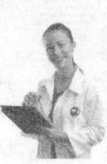

Food purchasing place: Market/local shop/weekly market places/others, specify _____

Household food production: No/vegetable garden/fruit tree/agriculture land/others, specify _____

Domestic animals: No/cow/buffalo/goat/pig/others, specify _____

Poultry: No/hen/duck/others, specify _____

Raw food preservation: No store/kitchen/store room/living room/others, specify _____

Cooked food preservation: No storage/kitchen/cup-board/refrigerator/others, specify _____

Type of cooking fuel: LPG/electric heater/kerosene stove/firewood/others, specify _____

Kitchen/cooking place: Clean/dirty _____

Number of meals per day _____

Anthropometric Measurement (In children)

Weight _____kg   Length/Height _____ cm   MAC_____cm   CC_____cm   HC_____cm

Degree of Malnutrition

Weight for Age $= \dfrac{\text{Actual weight of the child}}{\text{Expected weight of the child}} \times 100 =$ _____

Classification According to IAP

Weight for Age	Classification of under nutrition	In child
≥80%	Normal	Yes/No
71–80%	Grade-I	Yes/No
61–70%	Grade-II	Yes/No
51–60%	Grade-III	Yes/No
≤50%	Grade-IV	Yes/No

According to WHO Growth Charts

Weight for Age (0–3 Years)

Normal	Moderately Underweight (Below -2SD to 3SD)	Severely Underweight (Below 3SD)
Yes/No	Yes/No	Yes/No

Mid Arm Circumference (7 Months–60 Months)

<11.5 cm (Red)	11.5–12.5 cm (Yellow)	≥12.5 cm (Green)
Yes/No	Yes/No	Yes/No

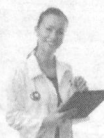

Anthropometric Measurement (In Adults)

Weight _____ kg   Height _____ cm

BMI (Quetelet's Index) _____   [Weight (kg)/height^2 (meter)]

Interpretation of BMI: Underweight/normal/overweight/obese

Family Dietary Pattern

Food group	Food item	Food consumption (yes/no)	Frequency of consumption (daily/ bi-weekly/ weekly/ monthly/ seasonally)	Average daily intake (in grams)	Expenditure per day (₹)	Method/Form of food preparation (boiling/steaming/ pressure cooking/ frying/baking/ germination/roasting/ fermentation)	Method of food storage at home (hygienic/ unhygienic)
Energy giving foods	Rice						
	Wheat						
	Tubers/roots						
	Edible oil						
	Ghee/butter						
	Dalda						
	Sugar/jaggery						
	Others						
Body building foods	Pulses						
	Meat						
	Fish						
	Poultry						
	Eggs						
	Others						
Protective foods	Vegetables						
	Fruits						
	Milk & milk products						
	Others						
Beverages	Tea						
	Coffee						
Others	Junk food						

PHYSICAL ASSESSMENT FOR COMMON NUTRITIONAL DEFICIENCIES

Site	Abnormal Signs	Possible Nutritional Deficiency	Remarks
Appearance	Thin/sick Obese	Undernutrition Overnutrition	
Growth	Low weight/stunted growth	Protein/Energy/Zinc	
Skin	Dry and scaly/flaky/rough Delayed wound healing Dermatitis	Vitamin A/Essential Fatty Acids Vitamin C Niacin	
Hair	Thin and sparse/dry/lusterless/ Depigmentation/easily pluckable	Protein/Energy	
Face	Pale Edema/moon face	Iron/Vitamin-B6/B-12/Folate Protein	
Eyes	Pale Night blindness/Bitot's spot/ xerophthalmia	Iron Vitamin-A	
Lips	Cracked around corners Swelling/puffiness	Iron/Riboflavin/Niacin/Vitamin-B6 Riboflavin/Niacin	
Tongue	Pale	Iron/Vitamin B-12/Folic Acid	
Teeth	Mottled enamel/dental caries Discoloration	Excess Sugar Intake/Poor Dental Hygiene Dental Fluorosis	
Gums	Swelling/bleeding	Vitamin C (Ascorbic Acid)	
Neck	Thyroid gland enlargement	Iodine (Goiter)	
Nails	Pale/spoon shaped/Brittle	Iron	
Muscles	Wasting	Protein/Energy	
Skeletal	Knock knees/bowed legs/pigeon chest/enlarged joints	Vitamin D/Calcium	

LAB INVESTIGATIONS

S. No.	Date/time	Investigation	Patient value	Normal Value	Remarks
		Hb Estimation Stool Examination Blood Smear			

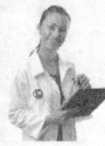

DIETARY PATTERN (24 HOURS RECALL)

Meal Time	Food item	Major Content	Quantity	Calories (kcal)	Carbohy-drate(g)	Protein (g)	Fat (g)	Iron (mg)	Calcium (mg)
Breakfast (__am)									
Midmorning (__am)									
Lunch (__pm)									
Evening Tea (__pm)									
Dinner (__pm)									
Bed time (__pm)									
Total									
Recommended Daily Values									
Deficient (–)/Excess (+)									

MODIFIED DIET PLAN

Meal Time	Food item	Major Content	Quantity	Calories (kcal)	Carbohy-drate (g)	Protein (g)	Fat (g)	Iron (mg)	Calcium (mg)
Breakfast (__am)									
Midmorning (__am)									
Lunch (__pm)									
Evening Tea (__pm)									
Dinner (__pm)									
Bed time (__pm)									
Total									
Recommended Daily Values									
Deficient (–)/Excess (+)									

Identified Health Problems/Needs

_____

_____

_____

_____

_____

_____

_____

_____

Prioritization of Health Problems/Needs

_____

_____

_____

_____

_____

_____

_____

_____

_____

Priority Nursing Diagnosis

_____

_____

_____

_____

_____

_____

_____

_____

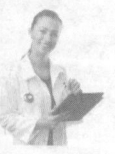

NURSING CARE PLAN

Assessment	Diagnosis	Goal/ Objective	Planning	Implementation	Evaluation

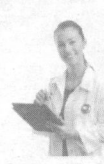

NURSING CARE PLAN

Assessment	Diagnosis	Goal/ Objective	Planning	Implementation	Evaluation

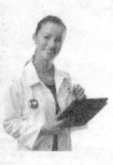

NURSING CARE PLAN

Assessment	Diagnosis	Goal/Objective	Planning	Implementation	Evaluation

HEALTH EDUCATION

(Include diet-selection/purchasing/cooking/serving/preservation/consumption/food hygiene/follow-up)

_____

_____

_____

_____

_____

_____

_____

_____

_____

_____

_____

_____

_____

_____

_____

_____

_____

REFERENCES

_____

_____

_____

_____

_____

_____

Signature of Student

Signature of Supervisor

GROWTH CHART – BOY (0-3 YEARS)

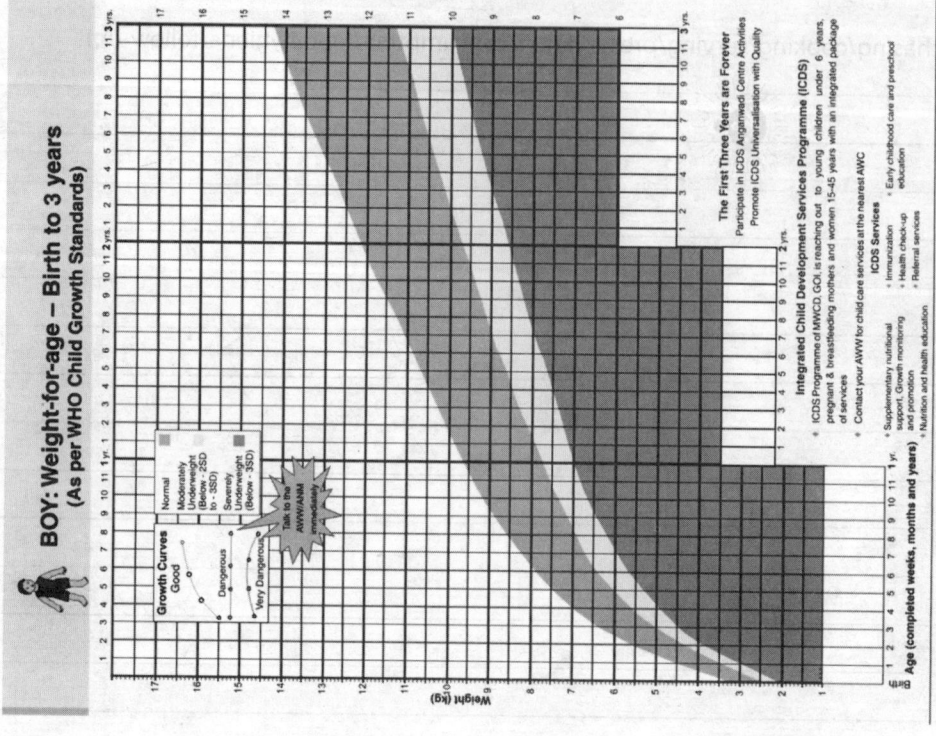

BOY: Weight-for-age – Birth to 3 years
(As per WHO Child Growth Standards)

The First Three Years are Forever
Participate in ICDS Anganwadi Centre Activities
Promote ICDS Universalisation with Quality

Integrated Child Development Services Programme (ICDS)
* ICDS Programme of MWCD, GOI, is reaching out to young children under 6 years, pregnant & breastfeeding mothers and women 15-45 years with an integrated package of services
* Contact your AWW for child care services at the nearest AWC

ICDS Services
* Supplementary nutritional support, Growth monitoring and promotion
* Nutrition and health education

* Immunization
* Health check-up
* Referral services

* Early childhood care and preschool education

Have your child weighed at the AWC every month

GROWTH CHART – GIRL (0-3 YEARS)

GIRL: Weight-for-age – Birth to 3 years
(As per WHO Child Growth Standards)

Diarrhoea
* Breastfeed more often
* Give extra fluids
* Give ORS & dispersible Zinc tablets as prescribed
* Continue feeding
* Take the child to hospital if loose motions do not stop

Fever
* If high fever take the child to the health centre

ARI
* If the child has rapid and/or difficult breathing, take the child to the health centre

+ Care During Illness +

Ensure equal care for the girl child

7. Nutritious Food Preparation/Cooking Demonstration

Name of the Recipe: _____

Name of the Client: _____

Age group/Age/Sex: _____

Diagnosis/Chief Complaints/Indication: _____

INTRODUCTION

_____

_____

_____

_____

OBJECTIVES

_____

_____

_____

_____

INGREDIENTS AND NUTRITIVE VALUE

Ingredient	Quantity	Calories (kcal)	Carbohydrate (g)	Protein (g)	Fat (g)	Iron (mg)	Calcium (mg)	Other important nutrients				
Total												

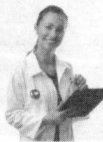

Price Calculation

S. No.	Ingredient	Price per kg Or per liter (₹)	Price as per amount used in Recipe (₹)
	Total		₹

Steps of Preparation

_____

_____

_____

_____

_____

_____

_____

_____

Health Education

_____

_____

Feedback

_____

_____

References

_____

_____

Signature of Student

Signature of Supervisor

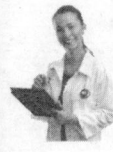

8. Bag Technique Procedure Demonstration

8.1. Vital Signs

IDENTIFICATION DATA

Name of the Student: _____

Date: _____

Name of the Client: _____

Age/Sex: _____

Chief Complaints: _____

Diagnosis: _____

Treatment (Taken/Not): _____

Student's Supervisor: _____

Definition

_____

_____

_____

Objectives/Need/Purpose

_____

_____

_____

Preparation of the Client

_____

_____

_____

Preparation of Articles

Article Name	Need/Purpose

Steps of Procedure

_____
_____
_____
_____
_____
_____
_____
_____
_____
_____
_____
_____
_____
_____
_____
_____
_____
_____

After Care of the Client

_____
_____
_____

After Care of the Articles

_____
_____
_____

Documentation

_____
_____
_____
_____

Signature of Student   **Signature of Supervisor**

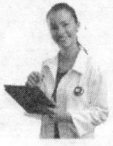

8.2. Urine Testing-Sugar/Albumin

IDENTIFICATION DATA

Name of the Student: _____

Date: _____

Name of the Client: _____

Age/Sex: _____

Chief Complaints: _____

Diagnosis: _____

Treatment (Taken/Not): _____

Student's Supervisor: _____

Definition

_____

_____

_____

Objectives/Need/Purpose

_____

_____

_____

Preparation of the Client

_____

_____

_____

Preparation of Articles

Article Name	Need/Purpose

Steps of Procedure

_____
_____
_____
_____
_____
_____
_____
_____
_____
_____
_____
_____
_____
_____
_____
_____
_____
_____
_____
_____
_____

After Care of the Client

_____
_____
_____

After Care of the Articles

_____
_____
_____

Documentation

_____
_____
_____
_____

Signature of Student   **Signature of Supervisor**

8.3. Collection of Specimen

8.3.1. Blood

IDENTIFICATION DATA

Name of the Student: _____

Date: _____

Name of the Client: _____

Age/Sex: _____

Chief Complaints: _____

Diagnosis: _____

Treatment (Taken/Not): _____

Student's Supervisor: _____

Definition

_____

_____

_____

Objectives/Need/Purpose

_____

_____

_____

Preparation of the Client

_____

_____

_____

Preparation of Articles

Article Name	Need/Purpose

Steps of Procedure

_____

_____

_____

_____

_____

_____

_____

_____

_____

_____

_____

_____

_____

_____

_____

_____

_____

_____

_____

_____

_____

After Care of the Client

_____

_____

_____

_____

After Care of the Articles

_____

_____

_____

Documentation

_____

_____

_____

_____

_____

Signature of Student   **Signature of Supervisor**

8.3.2. Sputum

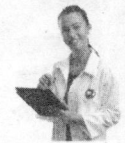

IDENTIFICATION DATA

Name of the Student: _____

Date: _____

Name of the Client: _____

Age/Sex: _____

Chief Complaints: _____

Diagnosis: _____

Treatment (Taken/Not): _____

Student's Supervisor: _____

Definition

_____

_____

_____

Objectives/Need/Purpose

_____

_____

_____

Preparation of the Client

_____

_____

_____

Preparation of Articles

Article Name	Need/Purpose

Steps of Procedure

_____
_____
_____
_____
_____
_____
_____
_____
_____
_____
_____
_____
_____
_____
_____
_____
_____
_____
_____

After Care of the Client

_____
_____
_____
_____

After Care of the Articles

_____
_____
_____
_____

Documentation

_____
_____
_____
_____

Signature of Student   **Signature of Supervisor**

8.3.3. Urine

IDENTIFICATION DATA

Name of the Student: _____

Date: _____

Name of the Client: _____

Age/Sex: _____

Chief Complaints: _____

Diagnosis: _____

Treatment (Taken/Not): _____

Student's Supervisor: _____

Definition

_____

_____

_____

Objectives/Need/Purpose

_____

_____

_____

Preparation of the Client

_____

_____

_____

Preparation of Articles

Article Name	Need/Purpose

Steps of Procedure

_____
_____
_____
_____
_____
_____
_____
_____
_____
_____
_____
_____
_____
_____
_____
_____
_____
_____
_____
_____
_____

After Care of the Client

_____
_____
_____
_____

After Care of the Articles

_____
_____
_____
_____

Documentation

_____
_____
_____
_____

Signature of Student   **Signature of Supervisor**

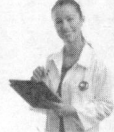

8.4. Hemoglobin Estimation

IDENTIFICATION DATA

Name of the Student: _____

Date: _____

Name of the Client: _____

Age/Sex: _____

Chief Complaints: _____

Diagnosis: _____

Treatment (Taken/Not): _____

Student's Supervisor: _____

Definition

_____

_____

_____

Objectives/Need/Purpose

_____

_____

_____

Preparation of the Client

_____

_____

_____

Preparation of Articles

Article Name	Need/Purpose

Steps of Procedure

_____
_____
_____
_____
_____
_____
_____
_____
_____
_____
_____
_____
_____
_____
_____
_____
_____
_____
_____
_____
_____
_____
_____

After Care of the Client

_____
_____
_____
_____

After Care of the Articles

_____
_____
_____
_____

Documentation

_____
_____
_____
_____

Signature of Student   **Signature of Supervisor**

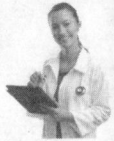

8.5. Malarial Parasite Slide Preparation

IDENTIFICATION DATA

Name of the Student: _____

Date: _____

Name of the Client: _____

Age/Sex: _____

Chief Complaints: _____

Diagnosis: _____

Treatment (Taken/Not): _____

Student's Supervisor: _____

Definition

_____

_____

_____

Objectives/Need/Purpose

_____

_____

_____

Preparation of the Client

_____

_____

_____

Preparation of Articles

Article Name	Need/Purpose

Steps of Procedure

_____

_____

_____

_____

_____

_____

_____

_____

_____

_____

_____

_____

_____

_____

_____

_____

_____

_____

_____

_____

_____

_____

_____

_____

After Care of the Client

_____

_____

_____

_____

After Care of the Articles

_____

_____

_____

_____

Documentation

_____

_____

_____

_____

Signature of Student   **Signature of Supervisor**

8.6. Oral Medication/DOTS

IDENTIFICATION DATA

Name of the Student: _____

Date: _____

Name of the Client: _____

Age/Sex: _____

Chief Complaints: _____

Diagnosis: _____

Treatment (Taken/Not): _____

Student's Supervisor: _____

Definition

_____
_____
_____

Objectives/Need/Purpose

_____
_____
_____

Preparation of the Client

_____
_____
_____

Preparation of Articles

Article Name	Need/Purpose

Steps of Procedure

_____
_____
_____
_____
_____
_____
_____
_____
_____
_____
_____
_____
_____
_____
_____
_____
_____
_____
_____
_____
_____

After Care of the Client

_____
_____
_____

After Care of the Articles

_____
_____
_____

Documentation

_____
_____
_____
_____

Signature of Student   **Signature of Supervisor**

8.7. IM/Subcutaneous Injection

IDENTIFICATION DATA

Name of the Student: _____

Date: _____

Name of the Client: _____

Age/Sex: _____

Chief Complaints: _____

Diagnosis: _____

Treatment (Taken/Not): _____

Student's Supervisor: _____

Definition

_____
_____
_____

Objectives/Need/Purpose

_____
_____
_____

Preparation of the Client

_____
_____
_____

Preparation of Articles

Article Name	Need/Purpose

Steps of Procedure

_____

_____

_____

_____

_____

_____

_____

_____

_____

_____

_____

_____

_____

_____

_____

_____

_____

_____

_____

_____

_____

_____

_____

After Care of the Client

_____

_____

_____

After Care of the Articles

_____

_____

_____

_____

Documentation

_____

_____

_____

Signature of Student   **Signature of Supervisor**

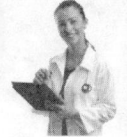

8.8. Drop Instillation

8.8.1. Ear Drop Instillation

IDENTIFICATION DATA

Name of the Student: _____

Date: _____

Name of the Client: _____

Age/Sex: _____

Chief Complaints: _____

Diagnosis: _____

Treatment (Taken/Not): _____

Student's Supervisor: _____

Definition

_____

_____

_____

Objectives/Need/Purpose

_____

_____

_____

Preparation of the Client

_____

_____

_____

Preparation of Articles

Article Name	Need/Purpose

Steps of Procedure

_____
_____
_____
_____
_____
_____
_____
_____
_____
_____
_____
_____
_____
_____
_____
_____
_____
_____
_____
_____
_____

After Care of the Client

_____
_____
_____
_____

After Care of the Articles

_____
_____
_____
_____

Documentation

_____
_____
_____
_____

Signature of Student   **Signature of Supervisor**

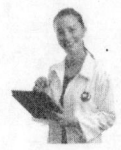

8.8.2. Eye Drop Instillation

IDENTIFICATION DATA

Name of the Student: _____

Date: _____

Name of the Client: _____

Age/Sex: _____

Chief Complaints: _____

Diagnosis: _____

Treatment (Taken/Not): _____

Student's Supervisor: _____

Definition

_____

_____

_____

Objectives/Need/Purpose

_____

_____

_____

Preparation of the Client

_____

_____

_____

Preparation of Articles

Article Name	Need/Purpose

Steps of Procedure

_____

_____

_____

_____

_____

_____

_____

_____

_____

_____

_____

_____

_____

_____

_____

_____

_____

_____

_____

After Care of the Client

_____

_____

_____

After Care of the Articles

_____

_____

_____

Documentation

_____

_____

_____

_____

Signature of Student   **Signature of Supervisor**

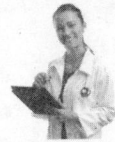

8.8.3. Nasal Drop Instillation

IDENTIFICATION DATA

Name of the Student: _____

Date: _____

Name of the Client: _____

Age/Sex: _____

Chief Complaints: _____

Diagnosis: _____

Treatment (Taken/Not): _____

Student's Supervisor: _____

Definition

_____
_____
_____

Objectives/Need/Purpose

_____
_____
_____

Preparation of the Client

_____
_____
_____

Preparation of Articles

Article Name	Need/Purpose

Steps of Procedure

_____
_____
_____
_____
_____
_____
_____
_____
_____
_____
_____
_____
_____
_____
_____
_____
_____
_____
_____
_____
_____

After Care of the Client

_____
_____
_____
_____

After Care of the Articles

_____
_____
_____

Documentation

_____
_____
_____
_____

Signature of Student

Signature of Supervisor

8.9. Breast Self-Examination

IDENTIFICATION DATA

Name of the Student: _____

Date: _____

Name of the Client: _____

Age/Sex: _____

Chief Complaints: _____

Diagnosis: _____

Treatment (Taken/Not): _____

Student's Supervisor: _____

Definition

_____

_____

_____

Objectives/Need/Purpose

_____

_____

_____

Preparation of the Client

_____

_____

_____

Preparation of Articles

Article Name	Need/Purpose

Steps of Procedure

_____
_____
_____
_____
_____
_____
_____
_____
_____
_____
_____
_____
_____
_____
_____
_____
_____
_____
_____
_____

After Care of the Client

_____
_____
_____
_____

After Care of the Articles

_____
_____
_____
_____

Documentation

_____
_____
_____
_____

Signature of Student   **Signature of Supervisor**

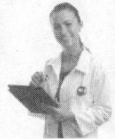

8.10. Testicular Self-Examination

IDENTIFICATION DATA

Name of the Student: _____

Date: _____

Name of the Client: _____

Age/Sex: _____

Chief Complaints: _____

Diagnosis: _____

Treatment (Taken/Not): _____

Student's Supervisor: _____

Definition

_____

_____

_____

Objectives/Need/Purpose

_____

_____

_____

Preparation of the Client

_____

_____

_____

Preparation of Articles

Article Name	Need/Purpose

Steps of Procedure

_____
_____
_____
_____
_____
_____
_____
_____
_____
_____
_____
_____
_____
_____
_____
_____
_____
_____
_____
_____
_____
_____

After Care of the Client

_____
_____
_____
_____

After Care of the Articles

_____
_____
_____
_____

Documentation

_____
_____
_____
_____

Signature of Student   **Signature of Supervisor**

8.11. Minor Wound Dressing

IDENTIFICATION DATA

Name of the Student: _____

Date: _____

Name of the Client: _____

Age/Sex: _____

Chief Complaints: _____

Diagnosis: _____

Treatment (Taken/Not): _____

Student's Supervisor: _____

Definition

_____

_____

_____

Objectives/Need/Purpose

_____

_____

_____

Preparation of the Client

_____

_____

_____

Preparation of Articles

Article Name	Need/Purpose

Steps of Procedure

_____
_____
_____
_____
_____
_____
_____
_____
_____
_____
_____
_____
_____
_____
_____
_____
_____
_____
_____
_____
_____
_____

After Care of the Client

_____
_____
_____
_____

After Care of the Articles

_____
_____
_____
_____

Documentation

_____
_____
_____
_____
_____

240

Signature of Student

Signature of Supervisor

8.12. Steam Inhalation

IDENTIFICATION DATA

Name of the Student: _____

Date: _____

Name of the Client: _____

Age/Sex: _____

Chief Complaints: _____

Diagnosis: _____

Treatment (Taken/Not): _____

Student's Supervisor: _____

Definition

_____

_____

_____

Objectives/Need/Purpose

_____

_____

_____

Preparation of the Client

_____

_____

_____

Preparation of Articles

Article Name	Need/Purpose

Steps of Procedure

_____

_____

_____

_____

_____

_____

_____

_____

_____

_____

_____

_____

_____

_____

_____

_____

_____

_____

After Care of the Client

_____

_____

_____

_____

After Care of the Articles

_____

_____

_____

_____

Documentation

_____

_____

_____

_____

Signature of Student

Signature of Supervisor

8.13. ORS Preparation

IDENTIFICATION DATA

Name of the Student: _____

Date: _____

Name of the Client: _____

Age/Sex: _____

Chief Complaints: _____

Diagnosis: _____

Treatment (Taken/Not): _____

Student's Supervisor: _____

Definition

_____
_____
_____

Objectives/Need/Purpose

_____
_____
_____

Preparation of the Client

_____
_____
_____

Preparation of Articles

Article Name	Need/Purpose

Steps of Procedure

_____
_____
_____
_____
_____
_____
_____
_____
_____
_____
_____
_____
_____
_____
_____
_____
_____
_____
_____

After Care of the Client

_____
_____
_____
_____

After Care of the Articles

_____
_____
_____
_____

Documentation

_____
_____
_____
_____

Signature of Student   **Signature of Supervisor**

8.14. Weaning

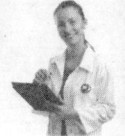

IDENTIFICATION DATA

Name of the Student: _____

Date: _____

Name of the Client: _____

Age/Sex: _____

Chief Complaints: _____

Diagnosis: _____

Treatment (Taken/Not): _____

Student's Supervisor: _____

Definition

_____

_____

_____

Objectives/Need/Purpose

_____

_____

_____

Preparation of the Client

_____

_____

_____

Preparation of Articles

Article Name	Need/Purpose

Steps of Procedure

_____
_____
_____
_____
_____
_____
_____
_____
_____
_____
_____
_____
_____
_____
_____
_____
_____
_____
_____
_____
_____

After Care of the Client

_____
_____
_____
_____

After Care of the Articles

_____
_____
_____
_____

Documentation

_____
_____
_____
_____

Signature of Student   **Signature of Supervisor**

8.15. Pediculosis Treatment

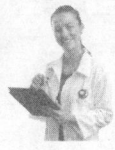

IDENTIFICATION DATA

Name of the Student: _____

Date: _____

Name of the Client: _____

Age/Sex: _____

Chief Complaints: _____

Diagnosis: _____

Treatment (Taken/Not): _____

Student's Supervisor: _____

Definition

_____
_____
_____

Objectives/Need/Purpose

_____
_____
_____

Preparation of the Client

_____
_____
_____

Preparation of Articles

Article Name	Need/Purpose

Steps of Procedure

_____
_____
_____
_____
_____
_____
_____
_____
_____
_____
_____
_____
_____
_____
_____
_____
_____
_____
_____
_____

After Care of the Client

_____
_____
_____
_____

After Care of the Articles

_____
_____
_____
_____

Documentation

_____
_____
_____
_____

Signature of Student   **Signature of Supervisor**

8.16. Hydrotherapy

IDENTIFICATION DATA

Name of the Student: _____

Date: _____

Name of the Client: _____

Age/Sex: _____

Chief Complaints: _____

Diagnosis: _____

Treatment (Taken/Not): _____

Student's Supervisor: _____

Definition

_____

_____

_____

Objectives/Need/Purpose

_____

_____

_____

Preparation of the Client

_____

_____

_____

Preparation of Articles

Article Name	Need/Purpose

Steps of Procedure

_____
_____
_____
_____
_____
_____
_____
_____
_____
_____
_____
_____
_____
_____
_____
_____
_____
_____
_____

After Care of the Client

_____
_____
_____
_____

After Care of the Articles

_____
_____
_____
_____

Documentation

_____
_____
_____
_____
_____

Signature of Student

Signature of Supervisor

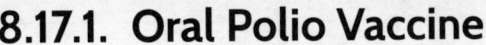

8.17. Immunization

8.17.1. Oral Polio Vaccine

IDENTIFICATION DATA

Name of the Student: _____

Date: _____

Name of the Client: _____

Age/Sex: _____

Chief Complaints: _____

Diagnosis: _____

Treatment (Taken/Not): _____

Student's Supervisor: _____

Definition

_____

_____

_____

Objectives/Need/Purpose

_____

_____

_____

Preparation of the Client

_____

_____

_____

Preparation of Articles

Article Name	Need/Purpose

Steps of Procedure

_____

_____

_____

_____

_____

_____

_____

_____

_____

_____

_____

_____

_____

_____

_____

_____

_____

_____

After Care of the Client

_____

_____

_____

After Care of the Articles

_____

_____

_____

Documentation

_____

_____

_____

_____

Signature of Student   **Signature of Supervisor**

8.17.2. Rotavirus Vaccine

IDENTIFICATION DATA

Name of the Student: _____

Date: _____

Name of the Client: _____

Age/Sex: _____

Chief Complaints: _____

Diagnosis: _____

Treatment (Taken/Not): _____

Student's Supervisor: _____

Definition

_____

_____

_____

Objectives/Need/Purpose

_____

_____

_____

Preparation of the Client

_____

_____

_____

Preparation of Articles

Article Name	Need/Purpose

Steps of Procedure

_____
_____
_____
_____
_____
_____
_____
_____
_____
_____
_____
_____
_____
_____
_____
_____
_____
_____
_____
_____
_____
_____

After Care of the Client

_____
_____
_____
_____

After Care of the Articles

_____
_____
_____
_____

Documentation

_____
_____
_____
_____

Signature of Student

Signature of Supervisor

8.17.3. Vitamin-A Administration

IDENTIFICATION DATA

Name of the Student: _____

Date: _____

Name of the Client: _____

Age/Sex: _____

Chief Complaints: _____

Diagnosis: _____

Treatment (Taken/Not): _____

Student's Supervisor: _____

Definition

_____

_____

_____

Objectives/Need/Purpose

_____

_____

_____

Preparation of the Client

_____

_____

_____

Preparation of Articles

Article Name	Need/Purpose

Steps of Procedure

_____

_____

_____

_____

_____

_____

_____

_____

_____

_____

_____

_____

_____

_____

_____

_____

_____

_____

After Care of the Client

_____

_____

_____

_____

After Care of the Articles

_____

_____

_____

_____

Documentation

_____

_____

_____

_____

Signature of Student

Signature of Supervisor

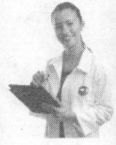

9. Preparation of A-V Aids

9.1. Charts

Introduction and Definition

_____
_____
_____
_____
_____

Objectives of Preparation

_____
_____
_____
_____
_____
_____

Principles

_____
_____
_____
_____
_____

Articles Required

S. No.	Name of the Article	Purpose	Quantity

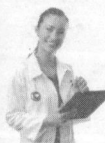

Budget Calculation

S. No.	Name of the Article	Source of Material (e.g. Market/household waste etc.)	Money Spent (₹)
	Total		₹

Steps of Preparation

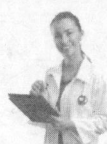

Paste a Picture/Draw a Diagram of Prepared A-V Aid

References

_____
_____
_____
_____
_____
_____
_____
_____
_____
_____
_____
_____
_____
_____
_____

Signature of Student

Signature of Supervisor

9.2. Flash Cards

Introduction and Definition

_____
_____
_____
_____
_____

Objectives of Preparation

_____
_____
_____
_____
_____

Principles

_____
_____
_____
_____
_____

Articles Required

S. No.	Name of the Article	Purpose	Quantity

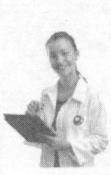

Budget Calculation

S. No.	Name of the Article	Source of Material (e.g. Market/household waste etc.)	Money Spent (₹)
	Total		₹

Steps of Preparation

_____

_____

_____

_____

_____

_____

_____

_____

_____

_____

_____

_____

_____

_____

_____

_____

_____

_____

_____

_____

_____

_____

_____

_____

Paste a Picture/Draw a Diagram of Prepared A-V Aid

References

Signature of Student

Signature of Supervisor

9.3. Model

Introduction and Definition

_____
_____
_____
_____
_____

Objectives of Preparation

_____
_____
_____
_____
_____
_____

Principles

_____
_____
_____
_____
_____

Articles Required

S. No.	Name of the Article	Purpose	Quantity

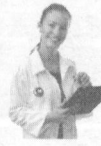

Budget Calculation

S. No.	Name of the Article	Source of Material (e.g. Market/household waste etc.)	Money Spent (₹)
	Total		₹

Steps of Preparation

Paste a Picture/Draw a Diagram of Prepared A-V Aid

References

Signature of Student

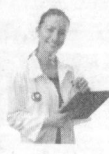

9.4. Pamphlet

Introduction and Definition

_____
_____
_____
_____
_____

Objectives of Preparation

_____
_____
_____
_____
_____
_____

Principles

_____
_____
_____
_____
_____

Articles Required

S. No.	Name of the Article	Purpose	Quantity

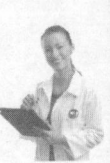

Budget Calculation

S. No.	Name of the Article	Source of Material (e.g. Market/household waste etc.)	Money Spent (₹)
	Total		₹

Steps of Preparation

_____

_____

_____

_____

_____

_____

_____

_____

_____

_____

_____

_____

_____

_____

_____

_____

_____

_____

_____

Paste a Picture/Draw a Diagram of Prepared A-V Aid

References

Signature of Student

Signature of Supervisor

9.5. Poster

Introduction and Definition

_____
_____
_____
_____
_____

Objectives of Preparation

_____
_____
_____
_____
_____
_____

Principles

_____
_____
_____
_____
_____

Articles Required

S. No.	Name of the Article	Purpose	Quantity

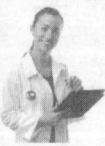

Budget Calculation

S. No.	Name of the Article	Source of Material (e.g. Market/household waste etc.)	Money Spent (₹)
	Total		₹

Steps of Preparation

Paste a Picture/Draw a Diagram of Prepared A-V Aid

References

_____
_____
_____
_____
_____
_____
_____
_____
_____
_____
_____
_____
_____
_____

Signature of Student   **Signature of Supervisor**

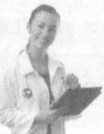

10. Participation in Activities/Clinics at SC/PHC/CHC/MCH Centers

10.1. Antenatal

INTRODUCTION

_____

_____

_____

_____

_____

Date: _____

Venue: _____

Time: _____

Distance from College (in km): _____

Type of Institution—Government/Private: _____

Name of the Student's Supervisor: _____

Objectives/Purpose: _____

_____

_____

_____

Equipment and Resources

S. No.	Equipment/Resources	Quantity	Source/Supply/Funding

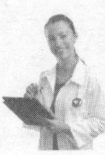

Health Personnel Involvement in Clinic/Camp Set-up

S. No.	Name of the Staff	Designation	Address of Hospital/Institute	Function

Steps/Method of Organizing Clinic/Camp

_____

_____

_____

_____

_____

_____

_____

_____

_____

Functions/Activities

_____

_____

_____

_____

_____

_____

_____

_____

_____

_____

273

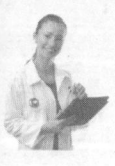

Map/Floor Plan Showing the Arrangement of Stations/Equipment/Resources at Clinic/Camp

Records and Reports Maintained

_____
_____
_____
_____
_____
_____
_____
_____
_____
_____

Student Nurse Learning

_____
_____
_____
_____
_____

Signature of Student   **Signature of Supervisor**

10.2. Postnatal

INTRODUCTION

_____
_____
_____
_____
_____
_____

Date: _____

Venue: _____

Time: _____

Distance from College (in km): _____

Type of Institution—Government/Private: _____

Name of the Student's Supervisor: _____

Objectives/Purpose: _____
_____
_____
_____
_____

Equipment and Resources

S. No.	Equipment/Resources	Quantity	Source/Supply/Funding

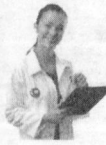

Health Personnel Involvement in Clinic/Camp Set-up

S. No.	Name of the Staff	Designation	Address of Hospital/Institute	Function

Steps/Method of Organizing Clinic/Camp

_____
_____
_____
_____
_____
_____
_____
_____
_____

Functions/Activities

_____
_____
_____
_____
_____
_____
_____
_____
_____

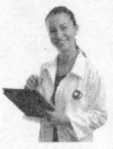

Map/Floor Plan Showing the Arrangement of Stations/Equipment/Resources at Clinic/Camp

Records and Reports Maintained

_____
_____
_____
_____
_____
_____
_____
_____
_____

Student Nurse Learning

_____
_____
_____
_____
_____

Signature of Student

Signature of Supervisor

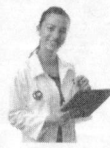

10.3. Family Welfare

INTRODUCTION

_____

_____

_____

_____

_____

_____

Date: _____

Venue: _____

Time: _____

Distance from College (in km): _____

Type of Institution—Government/Private: _____

Name of the Student's Supervisor: _____

Objectives/Purpose: _____

_____

_____

_____

_____

Equipment and Resources

S. No.	Equipment/Resources	Quantity	Source/Supply/Funding

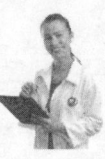

Health Personnel Involvement in Clinic/Camp Set-up

S. No.	Name of the Staff	Designation	Address of Hospital/Institute	Function

Steps/Method of Organizing Clinic/Camp

_____
_____
_____
_____
_____
_____
_____
_____

Functions/Activities

_____
_____
_____
_____
_____
_____
_____
_____
_____

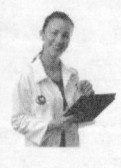

Map/Floor Plan Showing the Arrangement of Stations/Equipment/Resources at Clinic/Camp

Records and Reports Maintained

_____
_____
_____
_____
_____
_____
_____
_____
_____

Student Nurse Learning

_____
_____
_____
_____

Signature of Student   **Signature of Supervisor**

10.4. Under Five/Immunization

INTRODUCTION

_____

_____

_____

_____

_____

_____

Date: _____

Venue: _____

Time: _____

Distance from College (in km): _____

Type of Institution—Government/Private: _____

Name of the Student's Supervisor: _____

Objectives/Purpose: _____

_____

_____

_____

Equipment and Resources

S. No.	Equipment/Resources	Quantity	Source/Supply/Funding

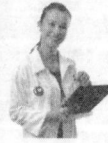

Health Personnel Involvement in Clinic/Camp Set-up

S. No.	Name of the Staff	Designation	Address of Hospital/Institute	Function

Steps/Method of Organizing Clinic/Camp

_____

_____

_____

_____

_____

_____

_____

_____

_____

Functions/Activities

_____

_____

_____

_____

_____

_____

_____

_____

_____

_____

Map/Floor Plan Showing the Arrangement of Stations/Equipment/Resources at Clinic/Camp

Records and Reports Maintained

_____

_____

_____

_____

_____

_____

_____

_____

_____

_____

Student Nurse Learning

_____

_____

_____

_____

Signature of Student   **Signature of Supervisor**

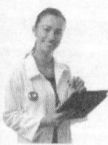

10.5. School Health

INTRODUCTION

_____

_____

_____

_____

_____

_____

Date: _____

Venue: _____

Time: _____

Distance from College (in km): _____

Type of Institution—Government/Private: _____

Name of the Student's Supervisor: _____

Objectives/Purpose: _____

_____

_____

_____

_____

Equipment and Resources

S. No.	Equipment/Resources	Quantity	Source/Supply/Funding

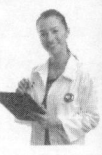

Health Personnel Involvement in Clinic/Camp Set-up

S. No.	Name of the Staff	Designation	Address of Hospital/Institute	Function

Steps/Method of Organizing Clinic/Camp

_____
_____
_____
_____
_____
_____
_____
_____
_____

Functions/Activities

_____
_____
_____
_____
_____
_____
_____
_____
_____
_____

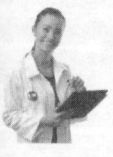

Map/Floor Plan Showing the Arrangement of Stations/Equipment/Resources at Clinic/Camp

Records and Reports Maintained

_____
_____
_____
_____
_____
_____
_____
_____
_____

Student Nurse Learning

_____
_____
_____
_____

Signature of Student

Signature of Supervisor

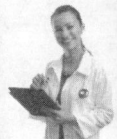

11. Community Health Survey

11.1. Mortality Survey

Name of the Survey Area _____ Date_____

DEATH IN THE FAMILY DURING THE LAST ONE YEAR

S. No.	Name	Age (yrs.) at death/ Sex	Occupation (Government/ Private/ homemaker/ unemployed)	Family Income per capita	Date of death	Place of death a) Government Hospital b) Private Hospital c) Home d) If other specify...	Reason for death a) Disease .... b) Accident .... c) If other specify	Death Registration in local authority a) Yes b) No
1.								
2.								
3.								
4.								
5.								
6.								
7.								
8.								

Survey Report

_____

_____

_____

Signature of Student   **Signature of Supervisor**

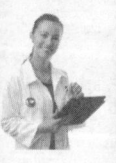

11.2. Morbidity Survey

Name of the Survey Area _____ Date _____

ANY ILLNESS IN THE FAMILY DURING LAST ONE YEAR

S. No.	Name	Age (yrs.)/ Sex	Education (a) Illiterate (b) Primary (c) Middle (d) Secondary (e) Senior secondary (f) Graduate (g) Above	Occupation (Government/ Private/ homemaker/ unemployed)	Family Income per capita	Diagnosis	Place of treatment (a) No treatment (b) Government Hospital (c) Private Hospital (d) If other specify___	Type of treatment (a) Allopathy (b) Ayurvedic (c) Homeopathy (d) Unani (e) Siddha (f) Naturopathy (g) If other specify___	Average money spent on treatment	Remarks
1.										
2.										
3.										
4.										
5.										
6.										
7.										
8.										
9.										
10.										

contd...

S. No.	Name	Age (yrs.)/ Sex	Education (a) Illiterate (b) Primary (c) Middle (d) Secondary (e) Senior secondary (f) Graduate (g) Above	Occupation (Government/ Private/ homemaker/ unemployed)	Family Income per capita	Diagnosis	Place of treatment (a) No treatment (b) Government Hospital (c) Private Hospital (d) If other specify____	Type of treatment (a) Allopathy (b) Ayurvedic (c) Homeopathy (d) Unani (e) Siddha (f) Naturopathy (g) If other specify____	Average money spent on treatment	Remarks
11.										
12.										
13.										
14.										
15.										
16.										
17.										
18.										
19.										
20.										

Survey Report

_____

_____

_____

Signature of Student

Signature of Supervisor

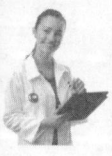

11.3. Family Planning Survey

Name of the Survey Area _____ Date _____

S. No.	Name of the eligible couple	Age (yrs.)/ Sex	Family Planning Practice (a) Yes (b) No (c) Yes, In the past	If yes, then Temporary Family Planning Method						Permanent Family Planning Method		Source of Family Planning method (a) Private Hospital (b) Government Hospital (c) If other specify ___	Duration of use (Months/ Years)	If No, then Willingness to adopt any contraceptive (a) Yes (b) No (c) Not decided	If yes, then name of the contraceptive to be adopted in future	Remarks
				Condom	Oral pills	Copper-T	Inject able	Implant	Tubectomy	Vasectomy						
1.																
2.																
3.																
4.																
5.																
6.																
7.																

contd...

S. No.	Name of the eligible couple	Age (yrs.)/ Sex	Family Planning Practice (a) Yes (b) No (c) Yes, In the past	If yes, then											If No, then		Remarks
				Temporary Family Planning Method						Permanent Family Planning Method		Source of Family Planning method (a) Private Hospital (b) Government Hospital (c) If other specify ___	Duration of use (Months/ Years)	Willingness to adopt any contraceptive (a) Yes (b) No (c) Not decided	If yes, then name of the contraceptive to be adopted in future		
				Condom	Oral pills	Copper-T	Inject able	Implant		Tubectomy	Vasectomy						
8.																	
9.																	
10.																	
11.																	
12.																	
13.																	
14.																	
15.																	

contd...

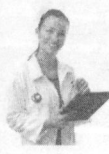

S. No.	Name of the eligible couple	Age (yrs.)/ Sex	Family Planning Practice (a) Yes (b) No (c) Yes, In the past	If yes, then										If No, then		Remarks
				Temporary Family Planning Method					Permanent Family Planning Method		Source of Family Planning method (a) Private Hospital (b) Government Hospital (c) If other specify ___	Duration of use (Months/ Years)	Willingness to adopt any contraceptive (a) Yes (b) No (c) Not decided	If yes, then name of the contraceptive to be adopted in future	
				Condom	Oral pills	Copper-T	Inject able	Implant	Tubectomy	Vasectomy					
16.															
17.															
18.															
19.															
20.															

Survey Report

_____

_____

Signature of Student   **Signature of Supervisor**

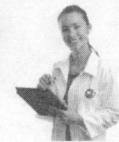

12. Practice Teaching

Lesson Plan On

_____

IDENTIFICATION DATA

Name of the Student Teacher: _____

Practice Teaching Topic: _____

Participants/Class/Group: _____

Size of the Group: _____

Date of Teaching: _____

Time of Teaching: _____

Duration of Teaching: _____

Place of Teaching: _____

Method of Teaching: _____

Teaching Aids: _____

Medium of Teaching/Language: _____

Name of the Student's Supervisor: _____

Self-Introduction

_____

_____

_____

_____

Topic Introduction

_____

_____

_____

_____

_____

_____

Previous Knowledge of the Group

_____
_____
_____
_____
_____

General Objective

_____
_____
_____
_____
_____

Specific Objectives

_____
_____
_____
_____
_____
_____
_____
_____
_____
_____
_____
_____
_____

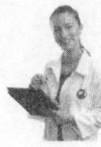

Time	Specific Objectives	Content	Health Educator Teaching Activity	A-V Aids	Participant's Evaluation

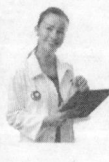

Time	Specific Objectives	Content	Health Educator Teaching Activity	A-V Aids	Participant's Evaluation

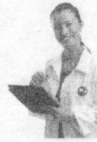

Time	Specific Objectives	Content	Health Educator Teaching Activity	A-V Aids	Participant's Evaluation

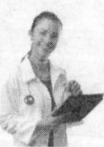

Time	Specific Objectives	Content	Health Educator Teaching Activity	A-V Aids	Participant's Evaluation

Time	Specific Objectives	Content	Health Educator Teaching Activity	A-V Aids	Participant's Evaluation

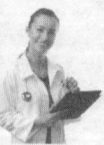

Time	Specific Objectives	Content	Health Educator Teaching Activity	A-V Aids	Participant's Evaluation

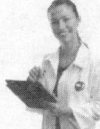

Time	Specific Objectives	Content	Health Educator Teaching Activity	A-V Aids	Participant's Evaluation

REFERENCES

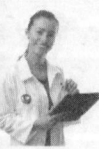

13. Group Project
(Role Play/Puppet Show/Exhibition/Health Camp)

INTRODUCTION

_____

_____

_____

_____

Schedule of Organization

- **Topic:** _____
- **Date:** _____
- **Venue:** _____
- **Time:** _____
- **Distance of Venue from the College (in km):** _____
- **Resource Person/Chief Guest:** _____
- **Beneficiaries:** _____
- **Name of the Student's Supervisor:** _____

Objectives

_____

_____

_____

_____

Articles/Equipments/Supplies Needed

S. No.	Name of the Articles/Equipment/Supplies	Purpose	Quantity

Budget Calculation

S. No.	Name of the Article	Money Spent (₹)
	Total	₹

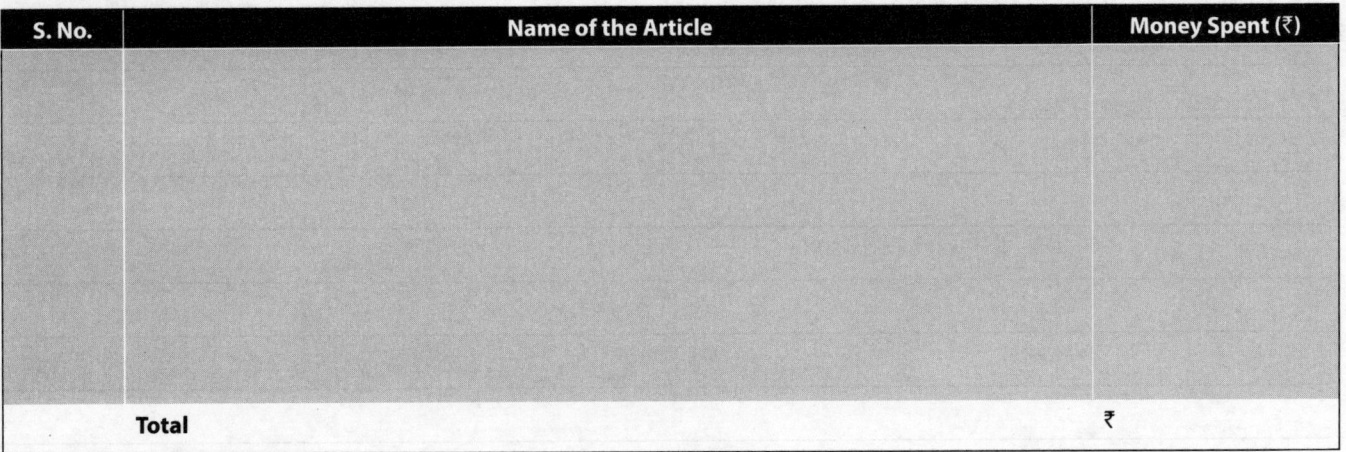

Source of Funding (College/Sarpanch/Doctors/Students/Others)

_____

_____

_____

_____

Steps of Organization of Group Project/Major Activities During the Group Project

_____

_____

_____

_____

_____

_____

_____

_____

_____

_____

_____

_____

_____

_____

_____

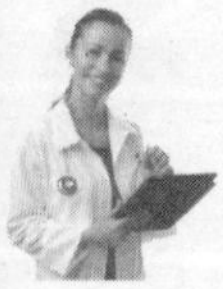

_____

_____

_____

_____

_____

_____

_____

_____

_____

_____

_____

_____

_____

_____

_____

_____

_____

_____

Paste the Pictures of Major Group Project Activities

(A)

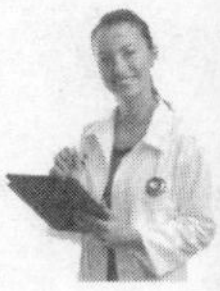

(B)

Feedback from the Beneficiaries

_____

_____

_____

_____

Student Nurse Learning from the Group Project

_____

_____

_____

_____

Signature of Student

Signature of Supervisor

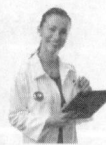

14. Observational Visits at Health and Welfare Agencies

14.1. Water Purification Plant

INTRODUCTION

_____

_____

_____

_____

Date: _____

Venue: _____

Time: _____

Distance from College (in km): _____

Name of the Head of the Water Purification Plant: _____

Type of Institution—Government/Private: _____

Name of the Student's Supervisor: _____

Visit Objectives

_____

_____

_____

_____

Organization Structure/Staffing Pattern

_____

_____

_____

_____

_____

Area Map/Physical Set-up (Floor Plan) of the Water Purification Plant   Keys

Components/Parts/Chambers

_____
_____
_____
_____

Procedure of Water Purification

_____
_____
_____
_____
_____
_____
_____

_____
_____
_____
_____
_____
_____
_____
_____
_____
_____
_____

Source of Funding

_____
_____
_____
_____

Records and Reports Maintained

_____
_____
_____
_____

Learning from the Visit for the Student Nurse

_____
_____
_____
_____

Signature of Student

Signature of Supervisor

14.2. Sewage Purification Plant

INTRODUCTION

_____
_____
_____
_____

Date: _____

Venue: _____

Time: _____

Distance from College (in km): _____

Name of the Head of Sewage Purification Plant: _____

Type of Institution—Government/Private: _____

Name of the Student's Supervisor: _____

Visit Objectives

_____
_____
_____
_____

Organization Structure/Staffing Pattern

_____
_____
_____
_____
_____
_____
_____
_____

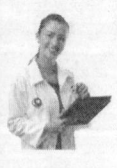

Area Map/Physical Set-up (Floor Plan) of the Sewage Purification Plant   Keys

Components/Parts/Chambers

_____

_____

_____

_____

Procedure of Sewage Purification

_____

_____

_____

_____

_____

_____

_____

_____
_____
_____
_____
_____
_____
_____
_____
_____
_____
_____
_____

Source of Funding

_____
_____
_____
_____

Records and Reports Maintained

_____
_____
_____
_____

Learning from the Visit for the Student Nurse

_____
_____
_____
_____

Signature of Student

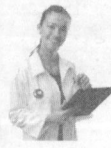

14.3. Infectious Disease Hospital

INTRODUCTION

_____

_____

_____

_____

Date: _____

Venue: _____

Time: _____

Distance from College (in km): _____

Name of the Head of the Institution: _____

Type of Institution—Government/Private: _____

Name of the Student's Supervisor: _____

Visit Objectives

_____

_____

_____

_____

Organization Structure/Staffing Pattern

_____

_____

_____

_____

_____

_____

_____

Physical Set-up (Floor Plan) of the Organization

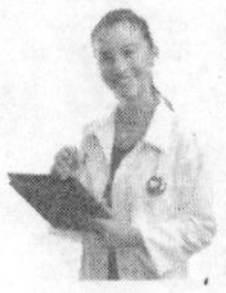

Departments/Areas Available

_____

_____

_____

_____

Source of Funding for the Organization

_____

_____

_____

Functions/Activities of the Organization

_____

_____

_____
_____
_____
_____
_____
_____
_____
_____
_____
_____
_____
_____

Beneficiaries of the Organization

_____
_____
_____
_____

Records and Reports Maintained in the Organization

_____
_____
_____
_____

Learning from the Visit for the Student Nurse

_____
_____
_____
_____

Signature of Student   **Signature of Supervisor**

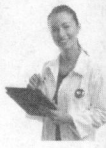

14.4. Factory/Occupational Health

INTRODUCTION

_____

_____

_____

_____

Date: _____

Venue: _____

Time: _____

Distance from College (in km): _____

Name of the Head of the Institution: _____

Type of Institution—Government/Private: _____

Name of the Student's Supervisor: _____

Visit Objectives

_____

_____

_____

_____

Organization Structure/Staffing Pattern

_____

_____

_____

_____

_____

_____

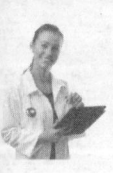

Physical Set-up (Floor Plan) of the Organization

Departments/Areas Available

_____

_____

_____

_____

Source of Funding for the Organization

_____

_____

_____

Functions/Activities of the Organization

_____

_____

_____
_____
_____
_____
_____
_____
_____
_____
_____
_____
_____
_____

Beneficiaries of the Organization

_____
_____
_____
_____

Records and Reports Maintained in the Organization

_____
_____
_____
_____

Learning from the Visit for the Student Nurse

_____
_____
_____
_____

Signature of Student

Signature of Supervisor

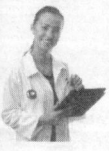

14.5. Old Age Home

INTRODUCTION

_____

_____

_____

_____

Date: _____

Venue: _____

Time: _____

Distance from College (in km): _____

Name of the Head of the Institution: _____

Type of Institution—Government/Private: _____

Name of the Student's Supervisor: _____

Visit Objectives

_____

_____

_____

_____

Organization Structure/Staffing Pattern

_____

_____

_____

_____

_____

_____

_____

Physical Set-up (Floor Plan) of the Organization

Departments/Areas Available

_____
_____
_____
_____

Source of Funding for the Organization

_____
_____
_____

Functions/Activities of the Organization

_____

_____

_____

_____

_____

_____

_____

_____

_____

_____

_____

Beneficiaries of the Organization

_____

_____

_____

_____

Records and Reports Maintained in the Organization

_____

_____

_____

_____

Learning from the Visit for the Student Nurse

_____

_____

_____

_____

Signature of Student

Signature of Supervisor

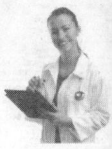

14.6. Non-Governmental Organizations (NGO)

INTRODUCTION

_____

_____

_____

_____

Date: _____

Venue: _____

Time: _____

Distance from College (in km): _____

Name of the Head of the Institution: _____

Type of Institution—Government/Private: _____

Name of the Student's Supervisor: _____

Visit Objectives

_____

_____

_____

_____

Organization Structure/Staffing Pattern

_____

_____

_____

_____

_____

_____

_____

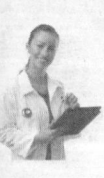

Physical Set-up (Floor Plan) of the Organization

Departments/Areas Available

_____

_____

_____

_____

Source of Funding for the Organization

_____

_____

_____

Functions/Activities of the Organization

_____

_____

_____

_____

_____

_____

_____

_____

_____

_____

_____

_____

Beneficiaries of the Organization

_____

_____

_____

_____

Records and Reports Maintained in the Organization

_____

_____

_____

_____

Learning from the Visit for the Student Nurse

_____

_____

_____

_____

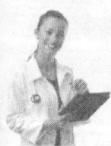

15. Home Visit and Family Folder

(Fill the family folders as per sample provided with the record book)

1. URBAN

Demographic Profile

Area: _____

Tehsil/Taluka: _____

Block: _____

District: _____

SC: _____

PHC: _____

CHC: _____

Family Folder Details

S. No	Date of issue	Name of head of the family	Address	Religion	Identified health needs	Interventions/ treatment	Date of submission	Signature of student	Signature of supervisor

2. RURAL

Demographic Profile

Area: _____

Tehsil/Taluka: _____

Block: _____

District: _____

SC: _____

PHC: _____

CHC: _____

Family Folder Details

S. No.	Date of issue	Name of head of the family	Address	Religion	Identified health needs	Interventions/treatment	Date of submission	Signature of student	Signature of supervisor

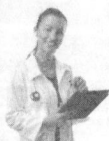

Annexures

NORMAL VALUES IN BLOOD INVESTIGATIONS

Blood investigations	Normal values
Hemoglobin	M: 13–17 g/dl FM: 11–15 g/dl
White Blood Cell count	4.0–10x10³/µL
WBC Differential Segmented neutrophils Band neutrophils Lymphocytes Monocytes Eosinophils Basophils	 50–70% 0–8% 20–40% 4–8% 0–4% 0–2%
Reticulocytes count	0.5–1.5% of RBC
Erythrocytes sedimentation rate (ESR)	<30 mm/hr
Hematocrit	M: 39–50% FM: 35–47%
Platelets (thrombocytes)	150–400 × 10³/µL
Bleeding time	2–7 min
Activated partial thromboplastin time (aPTT)	25–35 sec
Prothrombin time (PT)	11–16 sec
Red bold indices Mean corpuscular volume (MCV) Mean corpuscular hemoglobin (MCH) Mean corpuscular hemoglobin concentration (MCHC)	 80–100 fL 27–34 pg 32–37%
Blood urea	13–43 mg/dl
Serum creatinine	0.6–1.3 mg/dl
Serum Albumin	3.5–5.0 g/dl
Sodium	135–145 mEq/L
Potassium	3.5–5.0 mEq/L
Calcium	8.6–10.2 mg/dl
Cholesterol High-density lipoproteins (HDLs) Low-density lipoproteins (LDLs)	<200 mg/dl M:- >40 mg/dl Fe:- >50 mg/dl Recommended: <100 mg/dl
Bilirubin Total Indirect Direct	 0.2–1.2 mg/dl 0.1–1.0 mg/dl 0.1–0.3 mg/dl
Acetone Quantitative Qualitative	 <2.0 mg/dl Negative

contd…

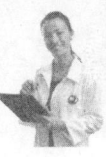

Blood investigations	Normal values
Ammonia	15–45 µgN/dl
Amylase	30–122 U/L
Lipase	31–186 U/L
Zinc	70–120 mcg/dl

NORMAL VALUES OF URINE INVESTIGATIONS

Urine investigations	Normal values
Acetone	Negative
Amylase	1–17 U/hr
Bilirubin	Negative
Calcium	100–250 mg/day
Creatine	<100 mg/day
Creatinine	0.6–2.0 g/day
Glucose	Negative
Hemoglobin	Negative
Ketone bodies	20–50 mg/day
Osmolality	300–1300 mOsm/kg
pH	4.0–8.0
Protein	0-trace
Sodium	40–220 mEq/day
Specific gravity	1.003–1.030
Uric acid	250–750 mg/day

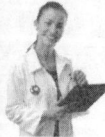

WHO RECOMMENDED NUTRITIVE VALUES FOR COMMONLY USED FOOD ITEM IN INDIA

Food Stuff	Amount	Proteins (g)	Fats (g)	CHO (g)	Energy (kcal)
Milk and Milk Products					
Milk toned	100 cc	3.5	3.5	5.0	66
Milk cow's	100 cc	3.2	4.1	4.4	67
Milk goat's	100 cc	3.3	4.5	4.6	72
Milk buffalo's	100 cc	4.3	6.5	5.0	117
Milk human	100 cc	1.1	3.4	7.4	65
Curds	100 cc	3.1	4.0	3.0	60
Curds toned	100 cc	3.0	3.0	4.0	55
Butter milk	100 cc	0.8	1.1	0.5	15
Milk powder	100 g	38.0	0.1	51.0	357
Milk liquid	100 cc	2.5	0.1	4.6	29
Paneer	100 g	18.3	20.8	1.2	265
Cheese processed	100 g	24.0	25.1	6.3	348
Whole milk powder	100 g	25.8	26.7	38.0	496
Cream	100 g	1.5	40.0	2.5	385
Cereals and Pulses					
Wheat atta	100 g	12.1	1.7	69.4	341
Rice	100 g	6.8	0.5	78.2	345
Maize	100 g	11.1	3.6	66.2	342
Gram	100 g	17.0	5.3	61.0	360
Porridge	100 g	12.0	1.5	71.2	346
Oat meal	100 g	13.6	7.6	62.8	37.4
Cornflakes	100 g	0.8	-	85.0	385
Popcorns (salt added)	100 g	13.0	5.0	87.0	385
Rice flakes	100 g	6.6	1.2	77.3	346
Rice puffed (salt added)	100 g	7.5	0.1	73.6	325
Suji	100 g	10.4	0.8	74.8	348
Vermicelli/Semiya	100 g	8.7	0.4	78.3	352
Maida	100 g	11.0	0.9	73.9	348
Corn flour or custard powder	100 g	0.5	-	86.6	345
Biscuit sweet	100 g	6.4	15.2	71.9	450
Bengal gram whole	100 g	17.1	5.3	60.9	360
Dal chana	100 g	20.8	5.6	59.8	372
Black gram dal	100 g	24.0	1.4	59.6	347
Urad dal washed	100 g	24.0	1.5	60.0	350
Green gram dal	100 g	24.5	1.2	59.9	348
Green gram whole	100 g	24.0	1.3	56.7	334
Lentil (masoor dal)	100 g	25.0	0.7	59.0	343
Red gram dal (Arhar)	100 g	22.3	1.7	57.6	335

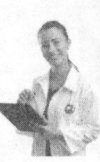

Food Stuff	Amount	Proteins (g)	Fats (g)	CHO (g)	Energy (kcal)
Peas dried	100 g	19.7	1.1	56.5	315
Rajma	100 g	23.0	1.3	60.6	346
Soya bean	100 g	43.2	19.5	20.9	432
Meat and Poultry					
Egg	100 g	13.3	13.3	-	173
Egg	One	6.6	6.6	-	76
Egg yolk	100 g	3.3	6.0	-	67
Egg white	100 g	3.0	-	-	12
Mutton (muscle)	100 g	18.5	13.3	-	194
Mutton (bone)	100 g	14.5	11.0	-	158
Fish	100 g	17.0	1.3	1.8	87
Chicken with bone	100 g	16.0	5.0	-	70
Chicken with muscle	100 g	25.0	0.5	-	109
Liver (goat)	100 g	20.0	3.0	-	107
Pork	100 g	18.7	4.4	-	114
Pigeon	100 g	23.3	4.9	-	137
Vegetables					
Cabbage	100 g	1.8	0.1	4.6	27
Coriander leaves	100 g	3.3	0.6	6.3	44
Curry leaves	100 g	6.1	1.0	18.7	108
Drum sticks	100 g	2.5	0.1	3.7	26
Fenugreek (methi)	100 g	4.4	0.9	6.0	49
Radish leaves	100 g	3.8	0.4	2.4	28
Lettuce	100 g	2.1	0.3	2.5	21
Mint	100 g	4.8	0.6	5.8	48
Mustard leaves (sarson)	100 g	4.0	0.6	3.2	34
Spinach	100 g	2.0	0.7	2.9	26
Carrot	100 g	0.9	0.2	10.6	48
Colocasia	100 g	3.0	0.1	21.1	97
Beet root	100 g	1.7	0.1	8.8	43
Onion	100 g	1.2	-	11.0	50
Onion small	100 g	1.8	0.1	12.6	59
Potato	100 g	1.6	0.1	22.6	97
Radish	100 g	0.7	0.1	3.4	17
Sweet potato	100 g	1.2	0.3	28.2	120
Turnip	100 g	0.5	0.2	6.2	29
Yam	100 g	1.4	0.1	26.0	111
Bitter gourd (karela)	100 g	1.6	0.2	4.2	25
Ghia	100 g	0.2	0.1	2.5	12
Brinjal	100 g	1.4	0.3	4.0	24
Cauliflower	100 g	2.6	0.4	4.0	30

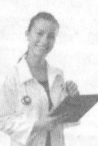

Food Stuff	Amount	Proteins (g)	Fats (g)	CHO (g)	Energy (kcal)
French beans	100 g	1.7	0.1	4.5	26
Giant chillies	100 g	1.3	0.3	4.3	24
Kholkhol	100 g	1.1	0.2	3.8	21
Lady finger	100 g	1.9	0.2	6.4	35
Peas	100 g	7.2	0.1	15.9	93
Pumpkin	100 g	1.4	0.1	4.6	25
Tinda	100 g	1.4	0.2	3.4	21
Tomato green	100 g	1.9	0.1	3.6	23
Tomato ripe	100 g	0.9	0.2	3.6	20
Cucumber	100 g	0.4	0.1	2.5	13
Fruits					
Apple	100 g	0.2	0.5	13.4	59
Amla	100 g	0.1	0.5	13.7	58
Apricot dried	100 g	1.6	0.7	73.4	306
Bael fruit	100 g	1.8	0.3	31.8	137
Banana	100 g	1.2	0.3	27.2	116
Apricot fresh	100 g	1.0	0.3	11.6	53
Cherries red	100 g	1.1	0.5	13.8	64
Currants black	100 g	2.7	0.5	75.2	316
Dates dried	100 g	2.5	0.4	75.8	317
Guava	100 g	0.9	0.3	11.2	51
Grapes	100 g	0.5	0.3	16.5	71
Lemon	100 g	1.0	0.9	11.1	57
Jamun	100 g	0.7	0.3	14.0	62
Litchie	100 g	1.1	0.2	13.6	61
Lime sweet (Musambi)	100 g	0.8	0.3	9.3	43
Mango	100 g	0.6	0.4	16.9	74
Orange	100 g	0.7	0.2	10.9	48
Orange juice	100 g	0.2	0.1	1.9	9
Papaya ripe	100 g	0.6	0.1	7.2	32
Peaches	100 g	1.2	0.3	10.5	50
Pear	100 g	0.6	0.2	11.9	52
Plums	100 g	0.7	0.5	11.1	52
Pineapples	100 g	0.4	0.1	10.8	46
Pomegranate	100 g	1.6	0.1	14.5	65
Raspberry	100 g	1.0	0.6	11.6	56
Nuts and Oil Seeds					
Almond	100 g	20.8	58.9	10.5	655
Cashew nuts	100 g	21.2	46.9	22.3	596
Charoli seeds	100 g	19.0	59.0	12.0	666
Coconut dry	100 g	6.8	62.3	18.4	662

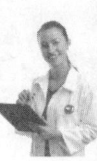

Food Stuff	Amount	Proteins (g)	Fats (g)	CHO (g)	Energy (kcal)
Coconut fresh	100 g	4.5	41.6	13.0	444
Walnut	100 g	15.6	64.5	11.0	687
Gingelly seeds	100 g	18.3	43.3	25.0	563
Ground nuts	100 g	26.2	39.8	26.7	570
Pistachio nut	100 g	19.8	53.5	16.2	626
Chilgoza	100 g	13.9	49.3	29.0	615
Butter and Oils					
Butter	100 g	-	81.0	-	729
Ghee (pure)	100 g	-	100	-	900
Vege cooking oil	100 g	-	100	-	900
Vanaspati ghee	100 g	-	100	-	900
Miscellaneous food stuff					
Arrowroot	100 g	0.2	0.1	83.1	334
Betel leaves	100 g	3.1	0.8	6.1	44
Cane sugar	100 g	0.1	0	99.4	398
Honey	100 g	0.3	0	79.5	319
Jaggery	100 g	0.4	0.1	95.0	383
Papped	100 g	18.8	0.3	52.4	288
Sago	100 g	0.2	0.2	87.1	351
Yeast dried	100 g	39.5	0.6	391	320
Jam	30 g	0.1	-	18.0	73
Beer 6%	250 cc	-	-	4.0	110
Whiskey 42%	50 cc	-	-	-	140
Brandy 54%	50 cc	-	-	-	150
Horlicks	One tb. spoon	2.4	0.1	7	42
Horlicks	100 g	14.0	0.8	72	416
Bread	100 g	7.8	0.7	52	245

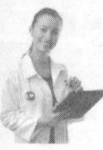

RECOMMENDED DIETARY ALLOWANCES (RDA) FOR VARIOUS CATEGORIES

Group	Particulars	Body wt. (kg)	Net energy Kcal/d	Protein g/d	Visible fat g/day	Calcium mg/day	Iron mg/d	Vitamin-A retinol	Vitamin-A β-carotene	Thiamine mg/day	Riboflavin mg/d	Niacin equivalent	Pyridoxine mg/d	Ascorbic acid mg/d	Dietary folate µg/d	Vit-B$_{12}$ µg/d	Magnesium mg/d	Zinc mg/day
Man	Sedentary work	60	2320		25					1.2	1.4	16						
	Moderate work	60	2730	60.0	30	600	17	600	4800	1.4	1.6	18	2.0	40	200	1.0	340	12
	Heavy work		3490		40					1.7	2.1	21						
Woman	Sedentary work	55	1900		20					1.0	1.1	12						
	Moderate work		2230	55.0	25	600	21	600	4800	1.1	1.3	14	2.0	40	200	1.0	310	10
	Heavy work		2850		30					1.4	1.7	16						
	Pregnant		+350	82.2	30	1200	35	800	6400	+0.2	+0.3	+2	2.5	60	500	1.2		
	Lactation 0-6 m		+600	77.9	30	1200	25	950	7600	+0.3	+0.4	+4	2.5	80	500	1.5		12
	6-12 m		+520	70.2	30					+0.2	+0.3	+3	2.5					
Infants	0-6 m	5.4	92 kcal/kg/d	1.16 g/kg/d	—	500	46 µg/kg/d	350	—	0.2	0.3	710 µg/kg	0.1	25	25	0.2	30	—
	6-12 m	8.4	80 kcal/kg/d	1.69 g/kg/d	19				2800	0.3	0.4	650 µg/kg	0.4				45	—
Children	1-3 years	12.9	1060	16.7	27	600	05	400	3200	0.5	0.6	8	0.9		80		50	5
	4-6 years	18.0	1350	20.1	25	600	09	600	4800	0.7	0.8	11	0.9		100	0.2-1.0	70	7
	7-9 years	25.1	1690	29.5	30		13	600	4800	0.8	1.0	13	1.6	40	120	0.2-1.0	100	8
Boys	10-12 years	34.3	2190	39.9	35	800	16	600	4800	1.1	1.3	15	1.6	40	140	0.2-1.0	120	9
Girls	10-12 years	35.0	2010	40.4	35	800	21			1.0	1.2	13	1.6	40	140	0.2-1.0	160	9
Boys	13-15 years	47.6	2750	54.3	45	800	27			1.4	1.6	16	2.0	40			165	11
Girls	13-15 years	46.6	2330	51.9	40	800	32	600	4800	1.2	1.4	14	2.0	40	150	0.2-1.0	210	11
Boys	16-17 years	55.4	3020	61.5	50	800	27			1.5	1.8	17	2.0	40			195	12
Girls	16-17 years	52.1	2440	55.5	35	800	28	600		1.0	1.2	14	2.0	40	200	0.2-1.0	235	12

Source: *Indian Council of Medical Research 2010*

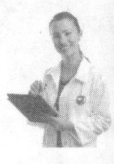

SUMMARY OF RECOMMENDED DIETARY ALLOWANCES (RDA) FOR ENERGY, PROTEIN, FAT AND MINERALS FOR INDIANS–2010

Group	Category/Age	Body weight (kg)	Net energy (kcal/kg/day)	Protein (g/kg/day)	Visible fat (g/day)	Calcium (mg/day)	Iron (mg/kg/day)	Zinc (mg/day)	Magnesium (mg/day)
Man	Sedentary work	60	2,320	60	25	600	17	12	340
	Moderate work		2,730		30				
	Heavy work		3,490		40				
Woman	Sedentary work	55	1,900	55	20	600	21	10	310
	Moderate work		2,230		25				
	Heavy work		2,850		30				
	Pregnant woman		+350	78	30	1,200	35	12	
	Lactation 0–6 months		+600	74	30	1,200	21		
	Lactation 6–12 months		+520	68	30				
Infants	0–6 months	5.4	92	1.16	–	500	46	–	30
	6–12 months	8.4	80	1.69	19		05	–	45
Children	1–3 years	12.9	1,060	16.7	27	600	09	5	50
	4–6 years	18.0	1,350	20.1	25		13	7	70
	7–9 years	25.1	1,690	29.5	30		16	8	100
Boys	10–12 years	34.3	2,190	39.9	35	800	21	9	120
Girls	10–12 years	35.0	2,010	40.4	35	800	27	9	160
Boys	13–15 years	47.6	2,750	54.3	45	800	32	11	165
Girls	13–15 years	46.6	2,330	51.9	40	800	27	11	210
Boys	16–17 years	55.4	3,020	61.5	50	800	28	12	195
Girls	16–17 years	52.1	2,440	55.5	35	800	26	12	235

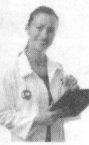

SOCIOECONOMIC SCALE

Socioeconomic Status Scales (India)

Rural	Udai Pareek , Modified BG Prasad, Shirpurkar, Radhuka
Urban	Modified Kuppuswamy Scale, Shrivastava, Jalota, Kulshreshtha, Gaurs

Table 1: Modified Kuppuswamy SOCIOECONOMIC STATUS Scale (India)

Education of head of family	Score
1. Professional degree or honors	7
2. Graduate or Postgraduate	6
3. Intermediate or Post High School Diploma	5
4. High School Certificate	4
5. Middle School Certificate	3
6. Primary School Certificate	2
7. Illiterate	1
Occupation of head of family	**Score**
1. Professional	10
2. Semi professional	6
3. Clerical, shop-owner, farmer	5
4. Skilled worker	4
5. Semi-skilled worker	3
6. Unskilled worker	2
7. Unemployed	1
Total monthly family income (in ₹- Using Consumer Price Index on Jan 2017)	**Score**
≥42259	12
21130–42258	10
15847–21129	6
10565–15846	4
6339–10564	3
2134–6338	2
≤2133	1
Total Score	**Socioeconomic class**
26–29	Upper (I)
16–25	Upper middle (II)
11–15 middle	Lower-middle (III)
5–10 lower	Upper-lower (IV)
< 5	Lower (V)

Minimum Score = 3, Maximum Score = 29

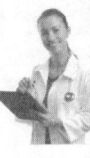

Table 2: Modified Pareek Rural Socioeconomic Status Scale

- Caste

  SC (1), Lower caste (2), Artisan caste (3), Agriculture caste (4), Prestige caste (5), Dominant caste (6).

- Occupation of head of family

  None (0), Laborer (1) Caste occupation (2), Business (3), Independent profession (4), Cultivation (5), Service (6)

- Education of head of family

  Illiterate (0), Can read only (1), Can read/write (2), Primary (3) Middle (4), High School (5), Graduate and above (6)

- Land holding

  No land (0), less than 1 acre (1), 1–5 acre (2), 5–10 acre (3), 10–15 acre (4), 15–20 acre (5), >20 acre (6).

- Social participation of head of family

  None (0), Member of one organization (like Panchayat, Nambardar etc.) (1), Member of >1 organization (2), Office holder in such organization (3), Wider public leader (6)

- Family Members up to 5 (1), Above 5 (2)

- Level of Housing

- No House (1), Kutcha House (2), Mixed House (3), Pucca House (4) Mansion (6)

- Farm Power

  No. drought (buffalo/cow) animal (1), 1–2 drought animal (2), 3–4 drought animals (3), 5–6 drought animals or tractor (6)

- Material Possession

  Bullock cart (1), Cycle (1), Radio (1), Chairs (1), Improved agriculture equipments (2), none (0)

Figures in () brackets indicate scores

Socioeconomic class [Pareek scale]	
Score more than 43	Class-I
Score 33–42	Class-II
Score 24–32	Class-III
Score 13–23	Class-IV
Score less than 13	Class-V

Table 3: BG Prasad Socioeconomic Scale

Socioeconomic class	Original classification (1960)–based on per capita family income in rupees	Updated based on per capita family in-come in rupees (2017)-method P Kumar
Class-I	100 and Above	6254 and Above
Class-II	50–99	3127–6253
Class-III	30–49	1876–3126
Class-IV	15–29	938–1875
Class-V	<15	<937

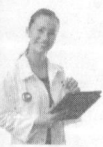

COMMUNITY NEED IDENTIFICATION AND VITAL STATISTICS SURVEY (PART-1)

General Information

Village/Area Name: _____

Panchayat: _____ Block: _____ Tehsil/Taluka: _____

District: _____

Total Population: _____

Total Families: _____

Fill the name of the organization and its distance from the community area in the space provided below

Nearby Health Care Facilities

District Hospital: _____

Government Maternity Hospital (if any): _____

Mission Hospital (if any): _____

Total Private Hospitals: _____

Sub Center: _____

Primary Health Center: _____

Community Health Center: _____

Indigenous medicine (hospital/clinic/dispensary)

- Ayurveda: _____
- Yoga: _____
- Naturopathy: _____
- Unani: _____
- Siddha: _____
- Homeopathy: _____
- If other, Specify: _____

Non-Governmental Organizations/Voluntary Health Organizations

- Orphan Age Children: _____
- Physically Challenged: _____
- Visually Challenged: _____
- Mentally Challenged: _____
- Hearing Challenged: _____
- Women: _____
- Elderly: _____
- Youth Welfare: _____
- Other: _____

Social Agencies

- Post Office: _____
- Bank: _____
- Police station: _____
- Facilities for the disposal of dead bodies _____

Religious Place
- Temple: _____
- Mosque: _____
- Gurudwara: _____
- Church: _____
- If others, Specify: _____

Education Facilities

Government
- Anganwadis: _____
- Balwadis: _____
- Primary School: _____
- Elementary School: _____
- Secondary School: _____
- Senior Secondary School: _____
- UG Institutions: _____
- PG Institutions: _____

Private
- Primary School: _____
- Elementary School: _____
- Secondary School: _____
- Senior Secondary School: _____
- UG Institutions: _____
- PG institutions: _____

Recreation Facilities
- Common Market Place: _____
- Playgrounds: _____
- Public Gardens: _____
- Cinema Halls: _____
- Clubs: _____
- Public Library: _____
- Fairs: _____
- Festivals: _____

Communication Facilities
- Post Office: _____
- Public Telephone Booths: _____
- Computer Center With Internet Facility: _____
- Traditional Media (Puppets, Folk Dance, etc.): _____

Transport Facilities
- Railway Station: _____
- Bus Stand: _____
- Auto Stand: _____
- Taxi Stand: _____
- Airport: _____

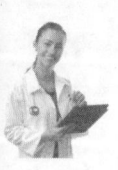

COMMUNITY NEED IDENTIFICATION AND VITAL STATISTICS SURVEY (PART-2)

Village/Area Name: _____ Tehsil/Taluka: _____ District: _____

2.1 SOCIO- DEMOGRAPHIC CHARACTERISTICS

General information			Age group							Sex			Religion					Caste				Marital Status			Type of family			Education								Occupation							
Family No.	Head of the family	Total family members	Family Member No.	Infant (1–12 months)	Under 5 (1–5 years)	School going (6–12 yr)	Adolescent (13–17 yr)	Early Adult (18–45 yrs.)	Late Adults (46–59 yrs.)	Geriatric (60 yr &above)	Male	Female	Transgender	Hindu	Muslim	Christian	Sikh	Others	General	OBC	SC	ST	Married	Unmarried/Single	Widow	Nuclear	Joint	Separated	Illiterate	Able to read and write	Primary	Secondary	Graduate	Post graduate	Others	Unemployed	Housewife	Govt. job	Private job	Retired	Daily wage worker	Total family income (₹)

2.2 HOUSING STANDARDS

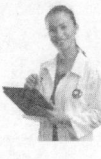

Family No.	Ownership of house		Type of house			No. of rooms in house	Bathroom					Latrine					Electricity		Water supply				Kitchen			Type of fuel used				
	Own	Rented	Pucca	Semi pucca	Kuccha		Not Available	Available		Hygiene		Not Available	Available		Hygiene		Available	Not available	Tap	Well	Lake/pond	Others	Separate	Corner of room	Others	LPG	Electricity	Kerosene	Wood	Others
								Own	Public	Hygienic	Unhygienic		Own	Public	Hygienic	Unhygienic														

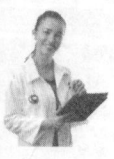

2.3 HOUSING ENVIRONMENT AND SANITATION

Family No.	Modern sanitation facility		Drainage system		Refuse disposal					Domestic animal (If present)						Cattle shed		Domestic birds/poultry (If present)			Poultry shed		Rodents (If present)		Insects (If present)				Street animals (If present)			
	Drainage system	Sewage system	Closed	Open	Open dumping	Composting	Burning	Community bins	Municipality collection	Dog	Cats	Buffalo	Cow	Goat	Others	Yes	No	Hen/cock	Parrot	Others	Yes	No	Rat	Others	Mosquitoes	Flies	Ticks	Others	Dogs	Cats	Cows	Others

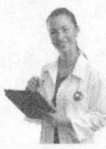

2.4 FAMILY PLANNING AND COMMON HEALTH PROBLEMS

Family No.	Total no. of eligible couple in the family	Total no. of women (15-49 years) in the family	Eligible Couple No./ Name	Method adopted for family planning								Family Member No.	Common health problems in last one year (Mention the number from the list given below)						Events within the last one year						
				Not using any method	Temporary methods					Permanent methods			Communicable disease *	Non- Communicable disease**	Nutritional problems***	Mental health problems #	Acute problems##	Chronic problems###	Any Birth	Any Death	Any neonatal death (infant less than 7 days)	Any neonate death (infant less than 28 days)	Any maternal death during antenatal, childbirth & postnatal period due to complications	Any still birth	Any infant death
					Condom	Oral pill	Copper-T	Injectable	Sub-dermal implants	Tubectomy	Vasectomy														

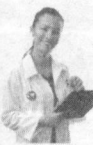

Common Health Problems

*Communicable disease –
1. Respiratory infection
2. Meningitis
3. Tuberculosis
4. Viral hepatitis
5. Diarrhea
6. Typhoid
7. Dengue
8. Malaria
9. Filaria
10. Viral infection
11. Others, specify_____

**Non-communicable disease –
1. Stroke
2. Anemia
3. Hypertension
4. Diabetes mellitus
5. Cardiovascular diseases
6. Cancer
7. Obesity
8. Others, specify_____

***Nutritional Problems-
1. Malnutrition
   (a) Over nutrition
   (b) Under nutrition
   (c) Other Nutritional deficiencies

*Mental Illness-
1. Depression
2. Mania
3. BPAD
4. Schizophrenia
5. OCD
6. Others, specify_____

**Acute Problems-
1. Cold
2. Cough
3. Pain
4. Inflammation/edema
5. Cut/bruises
6. Strain
7. Others, specify_____

***Chronic Problems-
1. COPD
2. Asthma
3. Rheumatic heart disease
4. Arthritis
5. Diabetes mellitus
6. Cancer
7. Hypertension
8. Others, specify_____

ANTHROPOMETRIC MEASUREMENTS

1. Weight

Average Birth-weight of Indian newborn is 2.7 to 2.9 kg .

Weight gain

In first 3 months = 25–30 g/month

Then up to 1 year = 400 g/month.

Note: In first 4–5 days after the birth, newborn babies loses their weight by 10%. From 10th day onwards, they regain their weight.

Usual weight gaining pattern

Age	Birth-weight
At birth	X
5 months	2X
1 year	3X
2 years	4X
3 years	5X
5 years	6X
7 years	7X
10 years	10X

Weight calculation

4-6 months = Birth-weight x 2

12 months = Birth-weight x 3

2 years = Birth-weight x 4

From 3–12 months = 1/2 (Age in months + 9) = Wt. in kg

1–6 years = Age in years x 2 + 8 = Wt. in kg

7–12 year = [Age in years x 7–5]/2 = Wt. in kg

For adult

According to Brocca Index

Expected weight = Height (in cm)-100 = Wt. in kg

2. Height

Usual height gaining pattern

Age	Length/height
At birth	50 cm
6 months	65 cm
1 year	75 cm
2 years	85 cm
3 years	95 cm
4 years	100 cm

Height calculation

From 2 to 12 years = Age (in years) x 6 + 77

After 4 years a child gains approximately 6 cm height every year until 12 years of age

3. Mid Arm Circumference (MAC)

Usual pattern of increase in mid arm circumference

Age	Mid arm circumference
At birth	11–12 cm
1 year	12–16 cm
1–5 years	16–17 cm
12 years	17–18 cm
15 years	20–21 cm

Classification of malnutrition (according to WHO)

Mid arm circumference	Grade
Above 13.5 cm	Normal
13.5–12.5 cm	Mild to Moderate(Grade-I and II)
Below 12.5 cm	Severe (Grade-III)

4. Head Circumference (HC)

It increases approximately 2 cm/month for first 3 months, 1 cm/month for next 3 months and 0.5 cm/month for rest of first year of life.

Usual pattern of increase in head circumference

Age	Head circumference
At birth	33–35 cm
3 months	40 cm
6 months	43 cm
2 years	48 cm
7 years	50 cm
12 years	52 cm
18 years	55 cm

Note: If there is 1 cm increase in head circumference in 2 weeks during first 3 months – Hydrocephalus is suspected.

5. Chest Circumference (CC)

Age	Chest circumference
At birth	2–3 cm less than Head Circumference (31–33 cm)
6–12 months	Both Chest Circumference and Head Circumference are equal
1 year	Chest Circumference >Head Circumference by 2.5 cm
5 years	Chest circumference is 5 cm >Head Circumference

6. Abdominal Circumference (AC)

Age	Abdominal circumference
At birth	32 cm

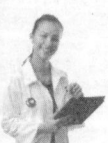

Family Folder (Sample Proforma)

Name and Address of Institute: _____

DEMOGRAPHIC PROFILE

Village/Area: _____ Tehsil/Taluka: _____ Block: _____

District: _____ SC: _____ PHC: _____ CHC: _____

FAMILY PROFILE

Name of Head of the Family: _____

Address: _____

_____

Religion—Hindu/Muslims/Sikh/Christian/Others: _____

_____

Caste—GEN/SC/ST/OBC: _____

Language known—Hindi/English/Others: _____

_____

Family Type—Nuclear/Joint: _____

Family Size (Total Members): _____

Ownership of House—Own/Rented: _____

Occupation of the head of the family—Unemployed/Government/Private Job/self-employed/daily wage worker/homemaker/others: _____

Total Monthly Family Income ₹: _____

Per Capita Family Income ₹: _____

FAMILY COMPOSITION AND CHARACTERISTICS

S. No.	Name of the family members	Relationship with head of the family	Date of Birth/Sex (Male-M/Female-F/Transgender-T)	Marital Status (Unmarried/Married)	Educational status	Occupation	Monthly income (₹)	Dietary habits (Veg/Non-veg)	Addiction (smoking alcohol/drugs/others)	Health status (Healthy/unhealthy)
1.										
2.										
3.										
4.										
5.										
6.										
7.										
8.										
9.										
10.										

HOUSING STANDARDS AND ENVIRONMENTAL CONDITIONS

Characteristic	Parameters
Type of house	Pucca/Semi pucca/Katcha
Site	Elevated from surroundings/depressed from surroundings
Total number of living room	1/2/3/4/5/6/7/8/ _____
Space per person	Adequate (1 room -2 persons, 2 rooms -3 persons, 3 rooms – 5 persons, 4 rooms -7 persons, 5 or more rooms - 10 persons (additional 2 for each further room Inadequate (if above criteria is not fulfilled)

contd...

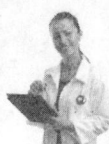

Characteristic	Parameters
Ventilation	Adequate (doors and windows facing each other in each room)
	Inadequate (doors and windows not facing each other in each room)
Bathroom	Not available/If available—Own/Public
Hygiene	Hygienic/Unhygienic
Wall	Plastered or Cemented/Tiled/Wooden/Unplastered/Mud//Others, specify _____
Roof	
Height	Less than 10 feet/More than 10 feet
Painting	Light colored/Dark colored
Day light	Adequate (Able to read the small fonts of newspaper inside the room during the day without any artificial lighting)
	Inadequate (Not able to read the small fonts of newspaper inside the room during the day without any artificial lighting)
Latrine	Not available/If available—Own/Public
Hygiene	Hygienic/Unhygienic
Electricity	Not available/Available
Drinking water supply	Tap/Well/Lake/Pond/Others, specify _____
Kitchen	Separate/Corner of the room/Others, specify _____
Type of fuel used	LPG/Electricity/Kerosene/Wood/Others, specify _____
Open space around the house	Absent/Present
Stagnant water around the house	Absent/Present
Street road	Tar/Cement/Mud/Others
Street light	Absent/Present
Modern sanitation facility	
Drainage system	Yes/No
Sewage system	Yes/No
Drainage System	Closed/Open
Refuse Disposal	Open dumping/Composting/Burning/Municipality collection/Community bins/Others, specify _____
Domestic animal	Absent/If present—Dog/Cow/Buffalo/Goat/Camel/Others, specify _____
Separate cattle shed (for the house with domestic animals)	Yes/No
Domestic birds/Poultry	Absent/If present—Hen/Cock/Parrot/Others, specify _____
Separate poultry shed/cage (for the house with domestic birds)	Yes/No
Rodents	Absent/If present—Rat/Others, specify _____
Street animals	Absent/If present—Dogs/Cats/Cows/Others, specify _____
Insect vectors	Absent/If present—Mosquitoes/Flies/Ticks/Others, specify _____

SOCIOECONOMIC STATUS

Social class/Socioeconomic status (according to rural/urban socioeconomic scale)

VULNERABLE/TARGET GROUPS IN THE FAMILY

Total eligible couples _____   Children (0–1 years) _____   Adolescent Girls _____

Total postnatal mothers _____   Children (1–3 years) _____   Elderly (above 60 years) _____

Total antenatal mothers _____   Children (3–5 years) _____   Other, specify _____

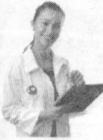

FAMILY DIETARY PATTERN

Food group	Food item	Food consumption (Yes/No)	Frequency of consumption (servings per day or per week)	Method/Form of food preparation (boiling/steaming/raw/ pressure cooking/ frying/germination etc.)	Method of food storage at home (Hygienic-H/ Unhygienic-U)
Energy giving foods	Rice				
	Wheat				
	Tubers				
	Edible oil				
	Ghee				
	Butter				
Body building foods	Meat				
	Fish				
	Poultry				
	Eggs				
	Pulses				
Protective foods	Vegetables				
	Fruits				
	Milk and milk products				
Beverages	Tea				
	Coffee				
	Water				
Others	Junk food				

FAMILY PLANNING STATUS (ELIGIBLE COUPLE)

S. No.	Name of the eligible couple (Mr. _____ Mrs_____)	Age (yrs.)/ Sex (Male-M Female-F)	Family planning practice Yes No	Temporary family planning method					Permanent family planning method		Month and year of adoption/ Duration of use
				Condom	Oral pills	Copper-T	Injectable	Implant	Tubectomy	Vasectomy	
1.											
2.											
3.											
4.											

IMMUNIZATION STATUS

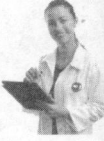

Age Group	Weeks/ Months/ Years	Current Vaccine Under UIP (2017)	Child Name/Vaccines/Date of administration (D.O.A.)					
			Child -1 _____		Child -2 _____		Child -3 _____	
			Vaccines	D.O.A.	Vaccines	D.O.A.	Vaccines	D.O.A.
Infant	At birth	BCG, OPV-0, Hep-B birth dose						
	6 weeks	OPV-1,Rota-1, Pentavalent-1, IPV-1, PCV-1						
	10 weeks	OPV-2,Rota-2, Pentavalent-2						
	14 weeks	OPV-3, Rota-3, Pentavalent-3, IPV-2, PCV-2						
	9 months	MR/Measles-1,Vit-A*, JE-1# PCV-Booster						
Under five Children	16–24 months	DPT-Booster-1, OPV-Booster, MR/Measles-2, JE-2#						
School Going	5–6 Years	DPT-Booster -2						
Adolescent	10 years	TT-1						
	16 years	TT-2						
Pregnancy		TT-1						
		TT-2						

*Vitamin A to be given every 6 months till five years of age and a separate chart is given below for documentation. #JE vaccine given in selected districts. **BCG:** Bacillus Calmette-Guerin**; Pentavalent [DPT:** diphtheria-pertussis-tetanus; **Hep B:** Hepatitis B; **Hib:**Haemophilus influenzae type b]; **JE:** Japanese Encephalitis; **MR/Measles/MMR:** Measles Mumps rubella; **OPV:** oral polio vaccine; **TT:** tetanus toxoid; **IPV:** inactivated poliovirus vaccine. **Rota-** Rotavirus vaccine, **PCV:** Pneumonia; Additional

Age (in months) →		9	18	24	30	36	42	48	54	60
Dose →		1st	2nd	3rd	4th	5th	6th	7th	8th	9th
Vitamin-A Solution (D.O.A.)	Child-1 _____									
	Child-2 _____									
	Child-3 _____									

FAMILY HEALTH ASSESSMENT AND DOMICILIARY CARE

Date/Time	Assessment	Nursing Intervention	Evaluation	Signature	
				Student	Supervisor

347

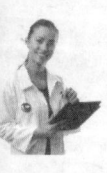

Woman Health Record

Name: _____

W/o: _____

Birth Year: _____

Husband: _____

Wife: _____

Educations Status

Age (in years)	15	16	17	18	19	20	21	22	23	24	25	26	27	28	29	30	31	32	33	34	35	36	37	38	39	40	41	42	43	44	45	46	47	48	49	50	51	52	53	54	Remarks
January																																									
February																																									
March																																									
April																																									
May																																									
June																																									
July																																									
August																																									
September																																									
October																																									
November																																									
December																																									

FULL COLUMNS WITH :

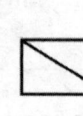

WEIGHT (In Kg.)

MENSES WITH DATE

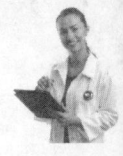

Antenatal Health Record

Obstetrics History

LMP	EDD	1st TT	2nd TT		
LMP	EDD	1st TT	2nd TT		

Date of Visit					
Weight					
Haemoglobin (Gm.)					
Blood Pressure					
Urine Sugar					
Urine Albumin					
Abdominal Girth					
Height of Uterus					
Foetal Position					
Foetal Heart Sound					
Engagement of Head					
Swelling on Face					
Swelling on Feet					
Giddiness					
Double Vision					
Breathlessness					

Remarks*	

Delivery Notes	Date : _____ Time : _____
Conducted by : _____	Place : _____
Delivery Notes	Date : _____ Time : _____
Conducted by : _____	Place : _____

* Prolapse Cord, Diminished or No foetal movements, Antepartum Haemmorrhage, Intranatal period, Postpartum Haemmorrhage

PREGNANCY		1	2	3	4	5	6	7	8	9	10
	Normal										
	Problem full term										
	Miscarriage										
	Abortion										
DELIVERY	Year										
	Month										
	Date										
	Time										
PLACE	Home										
	Hospital										
TYPE	Normal										
	Breech										
	Any other										
OUTCOME	Live Baby										
	Still Birth										
SEX	Male										
	Female										
PRESENT STATUS	Live										
	Dead										
If Dead, at what age :											
Birth Weight (In Kg.) :											
Conducted By :											

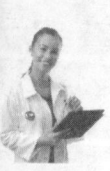

Post-natal Record

Educations Status : _____

Name: _____

Date of Delivery: _____   Address: _____

Date of Follow-up Visits : ⟶

Days (Age) ⟶	1	2	3	4	5	6	7	8	9	10	11	12	13	14	15	16	17	18	19	20	21	22	23	24	25	26	27	28	29	30	31	Remarks
1. Breast																																
- Engorgement																																
2. Nipples																																
- inverted/flat																																
- sore																																
- cracked																																
3. Perineum																																
- Episiotomy																																
- Tear																																
4. Discharge P/V																																
- Excessive																																
- Red																																
- Pink																																
- Creamish																																
- Foul Smelling																																
5. Personal Hygiene																																
- Dirty Clothes																																
- Perineal Clothes Unclean																																

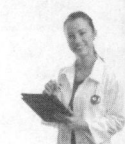

Date of Follow-up Visits : ——→

Days (Age) ——→	1	2	3	4	5	6	7	8	9	10	11	12	13	14	15	16	17	18	19	20	21	22	23	24	25	26	27	28	29	30	31	Remarks
6. Diet																																
- Liquid Milk Quantity																																
- Semisolid																																
- Extra Ghee																																
- Solid																																
7. Environment (Room)																																
- Unventilated																																
- Unclean																																
8. Treatment																																
- Hospital																																
- Private Doctors																																
- Home																																
- Any Other																																
9. Precaution from evil spirit																																

Remarks* ....

* Any abnormality - involution of uterus, Febrile condition
- Special Diet taken by mother - boiled water, Herbal Food, Ajwain, Special Food being Cooked

351

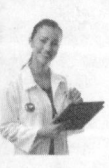

Newborn Health Record

Educations Status

Name: _____

Pet Name: _____

Sex: _____

Any Handicap

or abnormality: _____

Date of Follow Up Visits: →

Date of Birth: _____

Birth wt. (Within 24 hr) _____

Place of Birth: _____

Father's Name: _____

Mother's Name: _____

Birth Attendant's Name: _____

Designation: _____

Address: _____

Date: _____

House No.:: _____

Locality: _____

Days (Age) →	1	2	3	4	5	6	7	8	9	10	11	12	13	14	15	16	17	18	19	20	21	22	23	24	25	26	27	28	29	30	31	Remarks
Weight in Kg.																																
Illness																																
Fever																																
Cough																																
Running Nose																																
Distended abdomen																																
Pastules																																
Papules																																
Mosquitoes Bites																																
Rashes																																
Pneumonia																																
Diarrhoea																																
Oozing Cord Stump																																
Infected Cord Stump																																
Red Eyes																																
Discharge from Eyes																																
Others..............																																

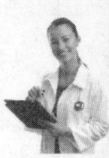

Date of follow up visits : ──→

Days (age) ──→	1	2	3	4	5	6	7	8	9	10	11	12	13	14	15	16	17	18	19	20	21	22	23	24	25	26	27	28	29	30	31	Remarks
Feeding																																
Breast feed																																
Ghutti																																
Sweat water																																
Salt water																																
Honey																																
Spoon feeding																																
Milk with spoon																																
Milk with bottle																																
Unable to take feed																																
Clothing																																
Clean																																
Seasonal																																
Clean bedding																																
Bathing by																																
Mother																																
Dai																																
Any other lady																																
Student																																
Treatment																																
Government doctor																																
Private doctor																																
Home remedy																																

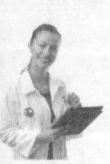

Child Health Record (Under Six)

Name: _____

Date of Birth: _____

Father's Name: _____

Birth wt.: _____

Sex M/F: _____

Month of Visit																																										
Age (in months)	01	02	03	04	05	06	07	08	09	10	11	12	13	14	15	16	17	18	19	20	21	22	23	24	26	28	30	32	34	36	38	40	44	48	52	56	60	64	68	72
N																																								
1																																								
2																																								
3																																								
4																																								

NUTRITIONAL HEALTH STATUS

Month and year of illness : Measles / Chicken Pox / Pneumonia / Mumps

Name of Vaccine	Date of Administration

Mile-stone Achieved

	Age (in months)
1. Sitting	
2. Crawling	
3. Standing without support	
4. Walking without support	
5. Completion of 4 incisors	
6. Clear use of 3 word sentences	
7. Drinking by self from glass	

Vitamin - A

1	2	3
4	5	6
7	8	9

Any Abnormality

Type of Feed	When Started	When Terminated
1. Colostrum		
2. Breast Feed		
3. Top Feed with		
- Bottle		
- Spoon		
4. Weaning		
5. Normal diet		

COMMUNITY PROFILE EVALUATION CRITERIA

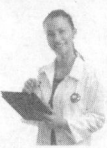

Name of the Area _____ Date: _____

Maximum Marks 30

S. No.	Particulars	Marks Allotted	Obtained Marks
1.	Introduction	2	
2.	Health Care/NGO/Social/Religious facilities	2	
3.	Educational/Recreation/Communication/Transport facilities	2	
4.	Sociodemographic Data	2	
5.	Physical Characteristics of Area (Map)	2	
6.	Housing Standards	2	
7.	Housing Environment and Sanitation	2	
8.	Family Planning Status	2	
9.	Common Health Problems	2	
10.	Vital Statistics	2	
11.	Ongoing Community Health Programmes	2	
12.	Ongoing Social Welfare/Health Schemes	2	
13.	List of Community Leaders	2	
14.	Identified Community Health Needs	2	
15.	Community Health Action Plan	2	
	Total	**30**	

Remarks

_____

_____

_____

_____

_____

_____

Signature of Supervisor

Date

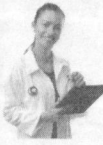

FAMILY CARE STUDY EVALUATION CRITERIA

Family Care Study On _____ Date: _____

Maximum Marks 50

S. No.	Particulars	Marks Allotted	Obtained Marks
1.	Introduction	2	
2.	Family Composition and Family Characteristics	2	
3.	Family tree/Family Genogramme	2	
4.	Health Care/Social/Educational Facilities	2	
5.	Recreation/Communication/Transport/Religious facilities	2	
6.	Sketch of House	1	
7.	Housing Standard and Environmental Conditions	1	
8.	Socioeconomic Status	1	
9.	Vulnerable/Target Groups	1	
10.	Family Budget	1	
11.	Family Dietary Pattern	1	
12.	Sociocultural Aspects	1	
13.	Family Planning Status	1	
14.	Immunization Status	1	
15.	Vital Events (Birth, Death, Marriage)	1	
16.	Family Health Profile	10	
17.	Book Picture (Comparison of Key case/s with Literature)	4	
18.	Health Need Identification/Prioritization/Nursing Diagnosis	4	
19.	Family Nursing Care Plan/Health Education	10	
20.	References	2	
	Total	**50**	

Remarks

_____

_____

_____

_____

_____

Signature of Supervisor

Date

FAMILY NURSING CARE PLAN EVALUATION CRITERIA

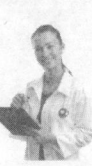

Family Nursing Care Plan On _____ Date: _____

Maximum Marks 50

S. No.	Particulars	Marks Allotted	Obtained Marks
1.	Introduction	2	
2.	Family Composition and Family Characteristics	2	
3.	Family tree/Family Genogramme	2	
4.	Health Care/Social/Educational Facilities	2	
5.	Recreation/Communication/Transport/Religious facilities	2	
6.	Sketch of House	1	
7.	Housing Standard and Environmental Conditions	1	
8.	Socioeconomic Status	1	
9.	Vulnerable/Target Groups	1	
10.	Family Budget	1	
11.	Family Dietary Pattern	1	
12.	Sociocultural Aspects	1	
13.	Family Planning Status	1	
14.	Immunization Status	1	
15.	Vital Events (Birth, Death, Marriage)	1	
16.	Family Health Profile	10	
17.	Health Need Identification/Prioritization/Nursing Diagnosis	4	
18.	Family Nursing Care Plan	12	
19.	Health Education	2	
20	References	2	
	Total	**50**	

Remarks

_____

_____

_____

_____

_____

Signature of Supervisor

Date

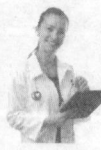

HEALTH ASSESSMENT EVALUATION CRITERIA

Health Assessment On: _____

Name of the Family Member: _____

Age/Sex: _____

Date: _____ Time: _____

Maximum Marks 40

S. No.	Particulars	Marks Allotted	Obtained Marks
1.	Identification Data	1	
2.	History Collection	2	
3.	Family Composition and Characteristics	2	
4.	Family tree/Genogramme	1	
5.	Housing Standard and Environmental Conditions	2	
6.	Physical Examination/Assessment Skill	8	
7.	Lab Investigations	2	
8.	Medications	2	
9.	Dietary Pattern (24 Hours Recall)	2	
10.	Modified Diet Plan	2	
11.	Health Need—Identification/Prioritization/Nursing Diagnosis	3	
12.	Family Nursing Care Plan	8	
13.	Health Education	3	
14.	References	2	
	Total	**40**	

Remarks

_____

_____

_____

_____

_____

Signature of Supervisor

Date

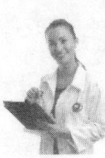

HEALTH EDUCATION EVALUATION CRITERIA

Health Education On: _____

Group: _____

Date: _____ Time: _____

Maximum Marks 30

S. No.	Particulars	Marks Allotted	Marks Obtained
1.	Selection of the Topic According to the Health/Group Need	2	
2.	Lesson Plan—Introduction	2	
3.	General and Specific Objectives	2	
4.	Content Relevant to the Topic	2	
5.	Content Adequacy and Sequence of Organization	2	
6.	Incorporation of Research Input/Current Trends/Issues	2	
7.	Summary and Conclusion	2	
8.	References	2	
9.	Classroom/Sitting Arrangement	2	
10.	Posture and Grooming (Neat and Tidy)	2	
11.	Communication Skills—Language, Voice Audibility, Clarity	2	
12.	Group Participation	2	
13.	Evaluation/Feedback	2	
14.	Appropriate Selection, Preparation and Use of A-V Aid	2	
15.	Time Coverage	2	
	Total	30	

Remarks

_____

_____

_____

_____

_____

Signature of Supervisor

Date

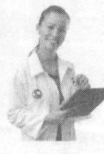

NUTRITIONAL ASSESSMENT (UNDER FIVE/ADULT) EVALUATION CRITERIA

Name of the Family Member: _____

Age/Sex: _____

Date: _____ Time: _____

Maximum Marks 30

S. No.	Particulars	Marks Allotted	Obtained Marks
1.	Identification data, Family Composition and Characteristics	2	
2.	Anthropometric Measurements (Including Growth Chart Plotting in Children)	4	
3.	Family Dietary Pattern	2	
4.	Assessment Skill for Common Nutritional Deficiencies	4	
5.	Lab Investigations	2	
6.	Individual Dietary Pattern (24 Hours Recall)	3	
7.	Modified Diet Plan	3	
8.	Health Need-Identification/Prioritization/Nursing Diagnosis	3	
9.	Family Nursing Care Plan	5	
10.	Health Education and References	2	
	Total	**30**	

Remarks

_____

_____

_____

_____

_____

_____

_____

_____

_____

_____

Signature of Supervisor

Date

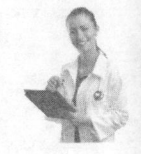

NUTRITIOUS FOOD PREPARATION/COOKING DEMONSTRATION EVALUATION CRITERIA

Cooking Demonstration On: _____

Name of the Family Member: _____

Age/Sex: _____

Date: _____ Time: _____

Maximum Marks 30

S. No.	Particulars	Good (3)	Average (2)	Poor (1)
1.	Develop the rapport with the family			
2.	Selection of demonstration according to nutritional need of the family member			
3.	Appropriate selection of ingredients and articles			
4.	Maintain hygiene (e.g. hand washing, cooking utensils)			
5.	Follow all the steps of preparation correctly			
6.	After care of the articles			
7.	Calculation of nutritive value			
8.	Calculation of price			
9.	Health education			
10.	Feed back from the family member			
	Total	30		

Remarks

_____

_____

_____

_____

_____

_____

_____

_____

Signature of Supervisor

Date

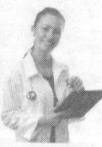

PROCEDURE EVALUATION CRITERIA

Bag Technique Procedure On _____ Date: _____

Maximum Marks 45

S. No.	Particulars	Good (3)	Average (2)	Poor (1)
1.	Develop the rapport with the family			
2.	Selection of procedure according to priority health need of the family			
3.	Preparation of community health bag according to the procedure			
4.	Follow bag technique correctly			
5.	Follow hand washing technique correctly			
6.	Preparation of the patient			
7.	Perform all the steps of procedure correctly			
8.	Carry out all the steps of procedure with scientific principles			
9.	Involvement of other family members in procedure			
10.	Communicate with patient and other family members while doing procedure			
11.	After care of the patient			
12.	After care of the articles and the community health bag			
13.	Dispose the waste correctly			
14.	Health education after the procedure			
15	Documentation of the procedure			
	Total	45		

Remarks

_____
_____
_____
_____
_____
_____
_____
_____
_____

Signature of Supervisor

Date

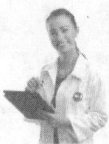

PREPARATION OF AUDIO-VISUAL AIDS EVALUATION CRITERIA

Topic: _____

Maximum Marks 20

S. No.	Particulars	Marks Allotted	Marks Obtained
1.	Plan for A-V aid preparation—Introduction, definition, objectives, principles, steps, layout, references	5	
2.	Principles followed	2	
3.	Budget calculation/Economical	2	
4.	Appropriate use of material and articles for model preparation	2	
5.	Accuracy/Size according to given dimensions	2	
6.	Utility	2	
7.	Simplicity	1	
8.	Solidity	1	
9.	Creativity	1	
10.	Submission on time	2	
	Total	**20**	

Remarks

_____
_____
_____
_____
_____
_____
_____
_____
_____
_____

Signature of Supervisor

Date

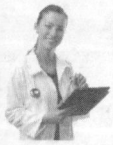

HEALTH ACTIVITY/CLINIC/CAMP EVALUATION CRITERIA

Health Activity/Clinic/Camp On_____

Date: _____ Time: _____

Place: _____

Maximum Marks 20

S. No.	Particulars	Marks Allotted	Obtained Marks
1.	Introduction/Objectives/Purpose	2	
2.	Arrangement of equipment and resources and their source	2	
3.	Health personnel involvement/their function	2	
4.	Map/floor plan showing arrangement of stations/equipment/resources	2	
5.	Organization of activities at different stations as per participant's need	2	
6.	Active participation in different activities of clinic/camp	2	
7.	Maintenance of record and report	2	
8.	Discipline/Time management	2	
9.	Evaluation and feedback from the participant	2	
10.	Student learning	2	
	Total	**20**	

Remarks

_____

_____

_____

_____

_____

_____

_____

_____

_____

Signature of Supervisor

Date

COMMUNITY HEALTH SURVEY EVALUATION CRITERIA

Community Health Survey On

_____

_____

Date: _____

Area: _____

Maximum Marks 40

S. No.	Particulars	Marks Allotted	Obtained Marks
1.	Introduction/Background/Literature Review	4	
2.	Need/Justification	4	
3.	Main objectives/sub-objectives	4	
4.	Methodology	4	
5.	Tool development	4	
6.	Data collection	4	
7.	Analysis and Interpretation	4	
8.	Result/Conclusion/Nursing Implementations/Recommendation	4	
9.	Discussion	4	
10.	References	4	
	Total	**40**	

Remarks

_____

_____

_____

_____

_____

_____

_____

_____

_____

Signature of Supervisor

Date

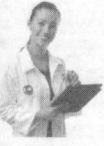

PRACTICE TEACHING EVALUATION CRITERIA

Practice Teaching On: _____

Group: _____

Date: _____ Time: _____

Maximum Marks 30

S. No.	Particulars	Marks Allotted	Marks Obtained
1.	Selection of the Topic According to the Health/Group Need	2	
2.	Lesson plan—Introduction	2	
3.	General and specific objectives	2	
4.	Content relevant to the topic	2	
5.	Content adequacy and sequence of organization	2	
6.	Incorporation of research Input/Current trends/Issues	2	
7.	Summary and Conclusion	2	
8.	References	2	
9.	Classroom/Sitting arrangement	2	
10.	Posture and Grooming (neat and tidy)	2	
11.	Communication skills—language, voice audibility, clarity	2	
12.	Group Participation	2	
13.	Evaluation/Feedback	2	
14.	Appropriate selection, preparation and use of A-V Aid	2	
15.	Time coverage	2	
	Total	30	

Remarks

_____

_____

_____

_____

_____

_____

Signature of Supervisor

Date

GROUP PROJECT EVALUATION CRITERIA

Group Project On: _____

Date: _____ Time: _____

Place: _____

Maximum Marks 20

S. No.	Particulars	Marks Allotted	Obtained Marks
1.	Introduction/Objectives/Purpose	2	
2.	Arrangement of equipment/resources and their purpose	2	
3.	Budget calculation	2	
4.	Source of funding	2	
5.	Organization of activities as per participant's need	2	
6.	Active participation in different activities of project	2	
7.	Maintenance of record and report	2	
8.	Discipline/Time management	2	
9.	Evaluation and feedback from the participant	2	
10.	Student Learning	2	
	Total	**20**	

Remarks

_____

_____

_____

_____

_____

_____

_____

_____

_____

Signature of Supervisor

Date

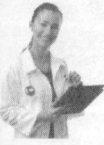

FAMILY FOLDER/HEALTH RECORD EVALUATION CRITERIA

Family Folder No: _____

Name of the Head of the Family: _____

Address: _____

Maximum Marks 10

S. No.	Particulars	Marks Allotted	Marks Obtained
1.	Clear	1	
2.	Accurate	1	
3.	Relevant	1	
4.	Completeness	1	
5.	Uniform writing style	1	
6.	Grammar/sentence formation	1	
7.	Up-to-date	1	
8.	Signed with date and time	1	
9.	Neat	1	
10.	Properly kept in folder cover or file	1	
	Total	**10**	

Remarks

_____

_____

_____

_____

_____

_____

_____

_____

_____

Signature of Supervisor

Date

OBSERVATION VISIT EVALUATION CRITERIA

Place of Visit: _____ Date: _____

Address: _____

Maximum Marks 20

S. No.	Particulars	Marks Allotted	Obtained Marks
1.	Introduction	2	
2.	Visit Objectives/Purpose	2	
3.	Organization Structure/Staffing Pattern	2	
4.	Lay out of Physical Set-up	2	
5.	Welfare Activities/Functions of Organization	2	
6.	Source of Funding/Budgeting	2	
7.	Record and Report Maintained	2	
8.	Student Participation in the Visit	2	
9.	Discipline/Time Management	2	
10.	Student's Learning from the Visit	2	
	Total	20	

Remarks

_____

_____

_____

_____

_____

_____

_____

Signature of Supervisor

Date

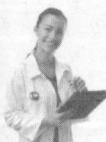

Suggested Readings

1. Santhi MV. Practical Record Book of Community Health Nursing –I. 1st edition. New Delhi:CBS Publisher and Distributors Pvt. Ltd; 2016.

2. Gulani KK. Community Health Nursing (Principles & Practices) 2nd edition. Delhi. Kumar Publishing House, 2005.

3. Singh MK. Complete Review of Preventive and Social Medicine. 2nd edition. New Delhi: CBS Publisher and Distributors Pvt. Ltd; 2016.

4. Park. K. Parks Text Book of Preventive and Social Medicine. 23rd edition: Jabalpur (MP). M/s Banarsidas Bhanot; 2015.

5. Taylor CR, Lillis C, LeMone P, Lynn P. Fundamentals of Nursing. The Art and Science of Nursing Care. 7th edition. New Delhi: Wolters Kluwer (India) Pvt. Ltd; 2012.

6. Sr. Nancy. Stephanie's Principles and Practice of Nursing. 6th edition. Indore (MP). NR Publishing House; 2016.

7. Rana AK, Saini SK. Practical Record Book of Midwifery. 1st edition. New Delhi: CBS Publisher and Distributors Pvt. Ltd; 2016.

8. Babu M, Gusain S. Clinical Case Record for Midwives. 4th edition. Delhi. Kumar Publishing House; 2009.

9. Government of India. Ministry of Health & Family Welfare. Guidelines for antenatal care and skilled attendance at birth by ANMs and LHVs-2010. [online] Available from: www.nhp.gov.in/sites/default/files/anm_guidelines. pdf [Assessed Sep 15, 2016]

10. Singh T et al. Socioeconomic status scales updated for 2017. Int J Res Med Sci. 2017;5(7):3264-3267 [online] Available from: www.msjonline.org [Assessed July 29, 2017]

11. Dutta P. Pediatric Nursing. 2nd edition. New Delhi: Jaypee Brothers Medical Publishers; 2009.

12. Sudhakar A. Practical Record Book of Child Health Nursing. 1st edition. New Delhi: CBS Publisher and Distributors Pvt. Ltd; 2016.

13. Gupta P. Clinical Methods in Pediatrics. 2nd edition. New Delhi: CBS Publisher and Distributors Pvt. Ltd; 2011.

14. Marlow DR, Redding BA. Textbook of Pediatric Nursing. South Asian edition. New Delhi. Elsevier India Private Limited; 2013.

15. World Health Organization. Guidelines for the implementation of the health promoting schools initiative (HPSI). Brazzaville-Congo: [online] Available from: URL: www.afro.who.int/[Assessed on 2012 Dec 12]

16. Nettina SM. Lippincott Manual of Medical and Surgical Nursing. 8th edition. New Delhi: Wolters Kluwer (India) Pvt Ltd; 2006.

17. Sharma R. Practical Record Book of Medical Surgical Nursing-II. 1st edition. New Delhi: CBS Publisher and Distributors Pvt. Ltd; 2016.

18. Singh R. Food and Nutrition for Nurses (B.Sc. Nursing). 1st edition. New Delhi: Jaypee Brothers Medical Publishers; 2012.

19. Budhwar S. A Textbook of Food and Nutrition for Nurses. 1st edition. Delhi. Kumar Publishing House, 2015.